THE **F*CK CANCER** *Cookbook*

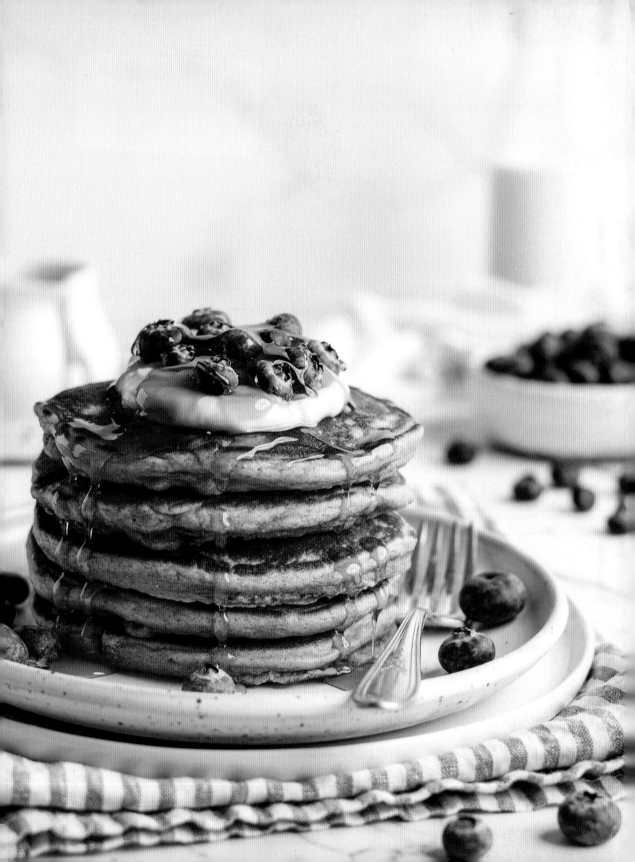

60 Nutrient-Dense and Holistic Recipes
for Taking Care of Your Body During and After Diagnosis

THE F*CK CANCER

Cookbook

Nichole Andrews

Oncology Registered Dietitian and Cancer Coach

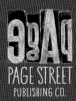

PAGE STREET
PUBLISHING CO.

PAGE STREET
PUBLISHING CO.

Copyright © 2023 Nichole Andrews

First published in 2023 by
Page Street Publishing Co.
27 Congress Street, Suite 1511
Salem, MA 01970
www.pagestreetpublishing.com

Distributed by Macmillan, sales in Canada by The Canadian Manda Group.

27   26   25   24   23   1   2   3   4   5

ISBN-13: 978-1-64567-834-2
ISBN-10: 1-64567-834-2

Library of Congress Control Number: 2022952206

Cover and book design by Meg Baskis for Page Street Publishing Co.
Lifestyle photography by Mark Cornellison
Food photography and styling by Amie MacGregor

Printed and bound in China

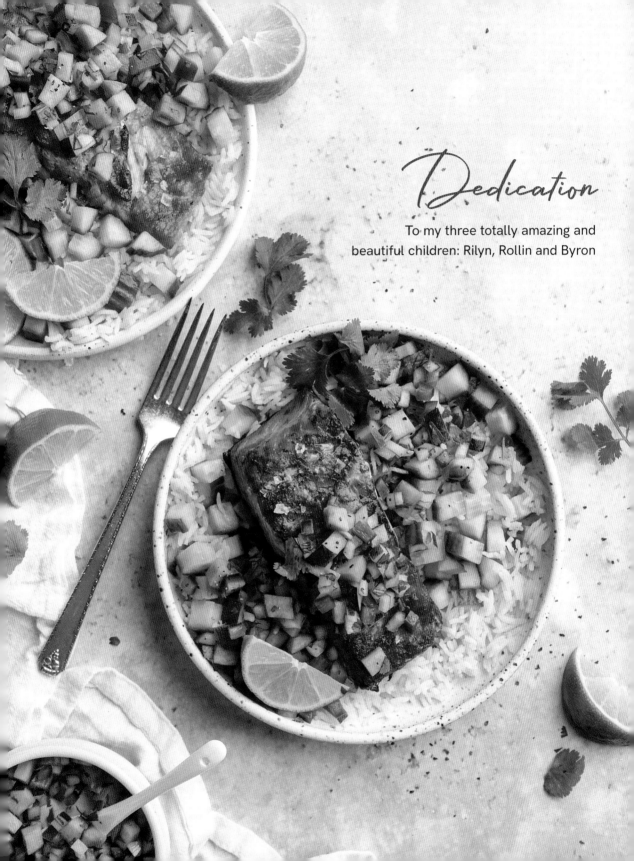

Dedication

To my three totally amazing and
beautiful children: Rilyn, Rollin and Byron

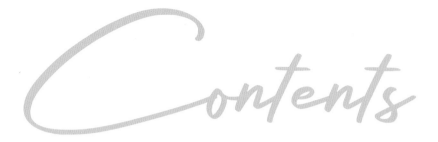

Contents

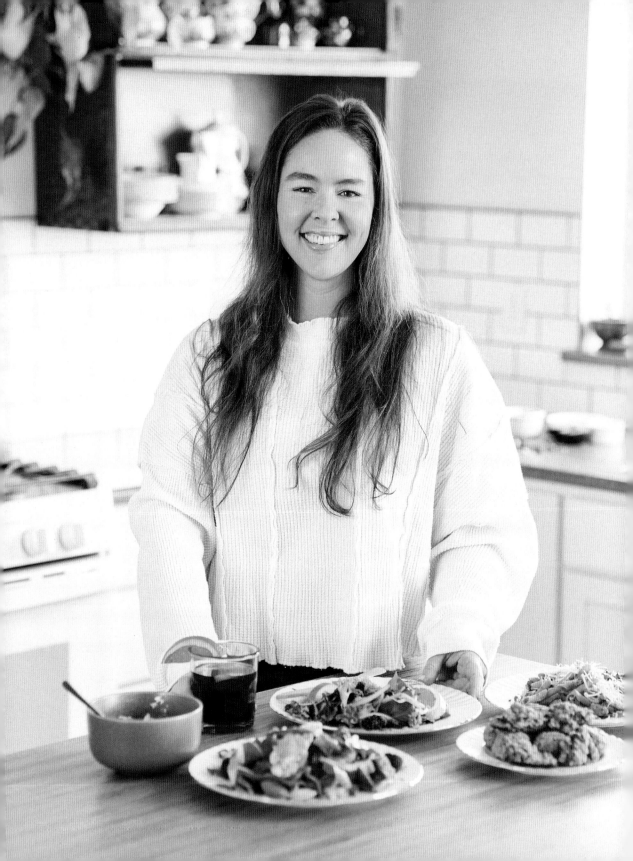

INTRODUCTION

Hi there! I'm Nichole, the Oncology Dietitian.

I'm an American Registered Dietitian (RD) specializing in oncology, and my passion is all about helping survivors both during and after cancer treatment to navigate the challenges of finding an eating routine that works for their individual health and cancer-prevention goals.

I know how hard you work as a cancer survivor. I know how ready and determined you are to be the healthiest version of yourself. In this book, I'll show you how to build meals and snacks to reduce cancer risk and make it feel easy. How many times have you read articles claiming that certain foods "feed" cancer or increase your cancer risk? It's terrifying. And it can make your favorite foods feel like they're off-limits—that's no way to live.

This book will help you understand how to BEST fuel your body to reduce cancer risk and to feel strong enough to fill your day-to-day life with the things that really count: fun, peace, quality family and friend time, alone time to recharge and social plans. Around here we fit cancer in around your life, not the other way around. You'll finally develop the strength to become untied from your recurrence or cancer-risk concerns.

With more than ten years' experience in oncology infusion, radiation, hormone therapy, pre- and post-op, survivorship and clinical and private practice, I can help you navigate this life-changing experience. Let's bust through all the misinformation out there and learn how to not only eat your food but enjoy it, too.

HOW TO START REDUCING YOUR CANCER RISK

Enjoying food and your meals is an important part of life—even when working toward a healthy lifestyle that reduces cancer risk. The great news is that you can do both of those things. I am going to share with you delicious and fun recipes that will also add nutritional value and reduce your cancer risk.

Nutrition has the power to reduce cancer risk, as our lovely foods contain macronutrients and micronutrients that work hard inside our bodies to keep cells strong, healthy and repaired daily! Thank you to those delicious foods!

How about the types of meat? Does one have to go vegan or vegetarian to reduce cancer risk? Nope! You still need protein to support a healthy lifestyle. So when having meat, dairy and eggs at each meal and/or snack, great choices are lean red meats (up to 18 ounces [510 g] a week and no more), turkey, chicken, seafood, fish, eggs and 1- to 2 percent- fat dairy. The only meat to eliminate is processed meat. Research suggests that regularly eating even small amounts of cold cuts, bacon, sausage and hot dogs increases colorectal cancer risk, which is why I recommend avoiding these foods as much as you can.

Is sugar really off-limits if you want to reduce cancer risk? Nope! Cancer is not caused by sugar. If you eat sugar, your cancer will not grow more quickly, just as if you were to omit it, cancer would not grow more slowly. You can limit sugary foods, as they are lower in nutrients and you do not want them to make up the majority of your food choices, but you do not have to remove them completely. That's not realistic or necessary, as most people enjoy such sweet treats as a soda at times, a rich dessert, a sweet snack, a slice of birthday cake or ice cream.

I am not advocating for a high-sugar diet, but you can still make a lot of room for a diet filled with all carbohydrates (fruit, grains, desserts and dairy—except cheese, as it is not considered a carbohydrate but rather, like other dairy prod-ucts, a protein), and have a part of that allotment be those sugary foods you love and want to enjoy throughout life, as most people do. Make sure to check out the dessert chapter (page 119) for recipe ideas! The more we restrict choices, the less control we can exert when we do eat them. And the more we focus on them, the more we want them, so we end up eating more of them than we planned. Allowing yourself to have them alongside your balanced diet of more plant-based foods, lean meats and lean dairy will help you curb any excesses!

What follows are proactive cancer-reducing steps that I want you to keep in mind. They encompass the areas we will focus on and, as with all recipes included in this book, will help you build a lifestyle that reduces cancer risk.

1. Add more plant-based foods to your diet and aim for 30 grams of fiber per day. The goal is to make all grains whole grains (or at least most of them) and to have 5 or more servings of a combination of fruits and vegetables per day. It's recommended that two-thirds of all your meals and snacks be made up of plant foods. These include beans, legumes, nuts, seeds, whole grains, fruits and vegetables. All are higher in fiber, which helps reduce cancer risk. Aim to get in 30 grams of fiber per day to reduce risk of breast and colon cancer. Eating more whole grains throughout your day will help you reach that goal.

2. Choose lean and plant protein options more often. These are safe choices to make to support a lifestyle that reduces cancer risk: chicken, turkey, dairy, eggs, fish and seafood. While reducing red meats (beef, pork and lamb) to no more than 18 ounces (510 g) per week, eliminate all processed meats, which increase the risk of colon cancer. Plant proteins that are good choices include chickpeas, edamame, quinoa, tofu and lentils.

3. Remove alcohol completely. Alcohol increases the risk of several cancers —breast, head and neck, esophageal and liver. Choosing non-alcoholic beverages more often will help you sleep better, have clearer cognition and lower your cancer risk.

4. Choose healthy fat options. Your body needs dietary fats daily. Dietary fats are essential for energy and to support cell function. They also help protect your organs and help keep your body warm. Fats help your body absorb certain nutrients and produce important hormones too. Consuming high levels of calories—regardless of the source—can lead to weight gain or being overweight. Consuming high levels of saturated or trans fats can lead to heart disease and stroke. Health experts generally recommend replacing saturated fats and trans fats with monounsaturated fats and polyunsaturated fats while still maintaining a nutritionally adequate diet. Some examples of healthy fats are soybean oil, corn oil, sunflower oil, olive oil, canola oil, peanut oil, safflower oil and sesame oil. Other sources include avocados, peanut butter and many nuts and seeds.

5. Choose lower-sodium options. If you are able to cut down on the amount of salt you eat, you can significantly reduce your risk of stomach cancer.

6. Limit sugary foods, sugary beverages and fast food. I want to make it clear that none of these foods are bad or have a direct link to increased risk of cancer, but they are lower in nutrition. You do not want the majority of your diet to be made up of sugar and fast foods: They are high in sugar, unhealthy fats and sodium. Drinking a lot of sugary drinks can contribute to weight gain, which increases your risk for cancer. So, instead of reaching for a soda, get into the habit of keeping some water or low-calorie beverages close by. Limiting processed food products helps you control your calorie intake and makes it easier to maintain a healthy weight.

7. There are only two things recommended that you eliminate to reduce your cancer risk. Alcohol and processed meats are the two items for which there is significant evidence showing they increase cancer risk. It's simply not part of a cancer-prevention lifestyle.

You have probably heard of a few caveats regarding increasing or reducing cancer risks, but I assure you most of those warnings and suggestions are myths. To make sure you know what I am talking about, let's do a lightning round of cancer nutrition myth busting to give you some relief and the ability to let these false recommendations go:

1. MYTH: Bread (or any carbs) are not safe, and you should go keto to treat or reduce risk of cancer.

    FACT: Don't go keto or remove major food groups to try to reduce cancer risk or as a magical cure: Carbs are needed to support your healthy cells and organs on a daily basis, not to mention to support your brain function, which will help limit cancer-induced brain fog.

2. MYTH: Sugar causes cancer.

    FACT: All our cells, cancerous or not, use glucose for energy. Our body doesn't pick and choose which cells get what fuel.

3. MYTH: Eat apricot seeds to cure cancer.

    FACT: There is currently no research to support the claim that apricot seeds can fight cancer. Furthermore, scientists have warned that a compound in the apricot kernel converts to cyanide in the body at levels that could be harmful.

4. MYTH: The only way to reduce cancer risk is to follow a vegan diet.

   FACT: Veganism is a personal choice, not the superior form of eating to reduce risk of cancer. Eating more plant foods helps to lower cancer risk, but you don't have to stick to just plant foods.

5. MYTH: You must juice to reduce risk of, or remove, cancer.

   FACT: Juices remove fiber, which you actually need more of to reduce risk; eat whole fruits/veggies or make smoothies to get all the protective components in plants.

6. MYTH: Acidic diets cause cancer.

   FACT: There's no good evidence to prove that diet can manipulate whole-body pH or that it has an impact on cancer. Your lungs and kidneys regulate your pH levels, so skip the notion that this diet is cancerous.

7. MYTH: Breast cancer survivors should avoid soy and flax.

   FACT: Major population studies show that eating soy does not increase a woman's risk for cancer recurrence, and it may even help reduce risk. These foods do not show harmful interaction with anti-estrogen medications.

8. MYTH: Superfoods prevent cancer.

   FACT: There's no such thing as a "superfood." It's a marketing term used to sell products and has no scientific basis. It's a gross oversimplification to say that any one food, on its own, could have a major influence over your chance of developing cancer.

9. MYTH: Taking a multivitamin lowers my cancer risk.

   FACT: Research suggests that taking a multivitamin or other supplement does not lower our cancer risk. In some cases, taking high doses of them has even been show to increase risk. Do not seek out extra supplements to try to reduce cancer risk—only take ones that your doctor has recommended to correct a deficiency that you cannot correct with food.

10. MYTH: There is a miracle cancer cure.

   FACT: YouTube videos and social media posts are emphatically not scientific evidence and aren't the same as good-quality, peer-reviewed evidence.

11. MYTH: Hormones in milk/meat cause cancer.

    FACT: There is no data to suggest that hormones present in milk can survive digestion or produce components that would have biological effects. Hormone receptors in humans do not recognize cow hormones and cannot produce effects in humans. Consuming dairy is linked to lowering colorectal cancer risk.

12. MYTH: Pesticides cause cancer, so you should eat organic.

    FACT: No studies have shown that people who consume organic foods have better health outcomes. Furthermore, organically grown produce is not entirely free of pesticides. Organic farmers use natural pesticides, whereas conventional farmers use synthetic pesticides. Neither designation—"natural" or "synthetic"—determines toxicity or the lack thereof. The determining factor is the dose, or amount, of the chemical that is ingested. Test results for both conventional and organic produce consistently show very low (and safe) levels of pesticide residue. Buy produce based on budget, smell and appearance, not on whether it is organic.

13. MYTH: Teflon pans cause cancer.

    FACT: The EPA does not indicate that the routine use of consumer products poses a concern. At present, there are no proven risks to humans from using cookware coated with Teflon.

14. MYTH: Leaving water bottles in your car will cause cancer.

    FACT: BPA is the chemical in question when it comes to the safe use of plastic. Use plastics as directed on the container label.

15. MYTH: Microwaves cause cancer.

    FACT: The rays in a microwave do not have enough power to damage DNA and therefore cannot cause cancer.

16. MYTH: Your body needs a "cleanse" to get rid of toxins that cause cancer.

    FACT: There is no scientific evidence that any "cleansing" products or procedures actually remove toxins in the body. Our liver and kidneys do that!

17. MYTH: Raw foods are more nutritious than cooked foods.

FACT: Some nutrients are deactivated during the cooking process, but some are activated. Consuming food items cooked and raw are both nutritious ways to eat.

18. MYTH: Artificial sweeteners cause cancer.

FACT: Current conclusions from well-designed studies do not show a clear causal relationship between artificial sweeteners and cancer.

19. MYTH: GMO foods cause cancer.

FACT: Current data can't confirm whether or not GMOs increase cancer risks. Consuming a diet rich in fruits, vegetables and whole grains outweighs any GMO health concerns when it comes to cancer risks.

In recent decades there has been a lot of evidence that supports changing lifestyle and nutrition to reduce risk of cancer. This is exciting, as anyone can (and should!) follow these recommendations to reduce risk and optimize their day-to-day food choices and routines throughout their life to live longer and feel good in their body.

When it comes to grocery shopping and picking out recipes that fit within a cancer-prevention lifestyle, there are a few main areas we will focus on: more plants, more whole grains, reducing processed meats and saturated fats, moderation of sugar and completely removing all alcohol.

Notice how we are mainly ADDING things to be healthier and reduce risk! That is what this cookbook is all about—amazing recipes with so many fun and flavorful ingredients you and your entire family can enjoy!

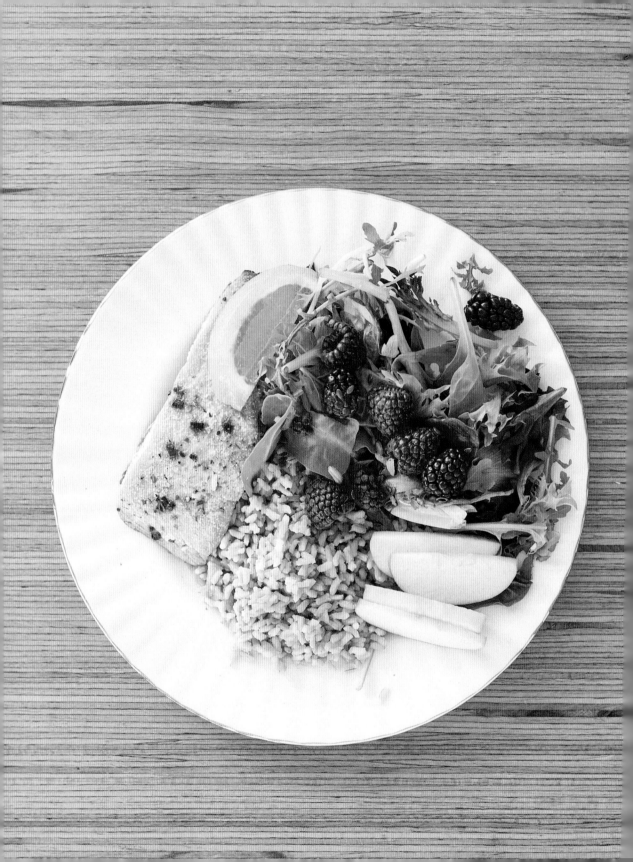

PLANT-FORWARD EATING FOR CANCER PREVENTION—SIMPLER THAN YOU THINK!

As your cancer dietitian, I want you to create a new plate method at meal and snack times. Oftentimes, typical home-cooked dinners are planned around a large portion of the meat, with some potatoes or other starchy vegetables on the side. Meals like these often contain too many calories and not enough health-protecting vitamins and minerals. Good news: It is easy to change this up but still keep your favorite foods (and recipes!)—in other words, to enjoy *all* foods and reduce cancer risk!

Plant-Forward Eating for Cancer Prevention:

- Two-thirds of your plate should contain plant foods (vegetables, fruits, whole grains, beans/legumes, nuts/seeds).
- One-third of your meals/snacks should include dairy, eggs, fish, poultry, meat, dessert and healthy fats.
- Limit/omit processed meats.
- Omit alcohol.
- Limit saturated fats.

WHAT IS A PLANT-FORWARD DIET?

A plant-forward diet is one that includes all foods except processed meats and alcoholic beverages. It is focused on two-thirds of the meals or snacks being made up of vegetables, fruits, whole grains, beans, legumes, nuts and/or seeds. Then the other one-third of the meal or snack is to be made up of fat sources, lean dairy, lean animal proteins and moderation of desserts. You do not have to go meatless or vegan to reduce cancer risk. Just focus on adding more plant foods with all meals and snacks.

These foods are rich in fiber, vitamins and other natural substances called phytochemicals, which help keep you in good health and protect against cancer. They are also naturally low in calories.

EAT THE RAINBOW TO REDUCE CANCER RISK!

Instead of painting a rainbow, how about eating a rainbow of colors? Red, orange, yellow, green, white, blue and purple.

Each of these colors has health benefits, including the following:

- Reduced risk of chronic diseases, including cancer, heart disease and diabetes
- Improved vision
- Decreased inflammation
- Strengthened immune system

The benefits are derived from the phytochemicals that occur naturally within these foods. Phytochemicals also give foods their distinct aroma and taste.

While each color provides certain benefits, when paired with other colors, the effects on your health are astonishing.

The cancer-protective benefits of adding more plant foods to your diet include the following:

- Fruits and vegetables protect against cancers of the mouth, pharynx, larynx, esophagus, stomach and lungs.
- Garlic, onions and leeks protect against stomach cancer.
- All foods that contain fiber reduce risk for colorectal cancer.
- Whole grain consumption protects against colorectal cancer.
- All plant foods are rich in phytochemicals, vitamins and minerals that work together to protect against all cancers.
- Selenium (found in cruciferous veggies: cabbage, broccoli and cauliflower) and lycopene-containing foods (watermelon, pink grapefruit, pink guava and papaya) protect against prostate cancer.
- Foods containing vitamin C and beta-carotene (often produce that is yellow, orange or green)—leafy fruits and vegetables such as carrots, spinach, lettuce, tomatoes, sweet potatoes, broccoli, cantaloupe and winter squash—protect against esophageal cancer.
- Foods that supply carotenoids, such as dark green and orange vegetables and fruits, help protect against cancer of the mouth, pharynx, larynx and lung.
- High-fiber intakes have been associated with lower breast cancer risk (as a general guideline, aim for 30 grams of fiber per day).

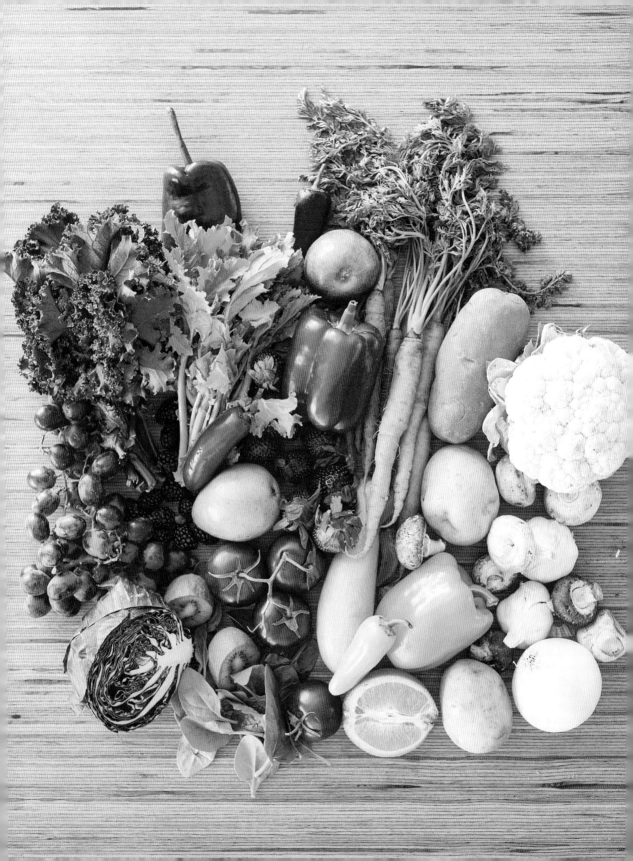

These food components have protective effects to slow the production of cancer cells through multiple mechanisms, such as apoptosis (cell death of unhealthy cells), DNA repair, hormone regulation and inflammatory responses.

For example, antioxidants (found in fruits and vegetables) protect against oxidative damage. Folate, which is found in legumes, leafy greens, nuts, seeds and broccoli, supports DNA repair. Selenium, which can be found in beans, lentils and mushrooms, protects from DNA damage and supports DNA repair. These are just a few examples of the amazing properties found in these protective plant foods!

THE DIFFERENCE BETWEEN ANTIOXIDANTS AND PHYTOCHEMICALS

Antioxidants: Substances that prevent damage to cells from highly reactive, unstable molecules called "free radicals." Antioxidants stabilize the free radicals. If not kept in check, free radicals lead to cell damage linked to various chronic diseases.

Phytochemicals: Naturally occurring compounds in plant foods such as fruits, vegetables, whole grains, beans, nuts and seeds. Phytochemicals neutralize free radicals and remove their power to create damage; many phytochemicals act as antioxidants.

When you consume foods to obtain those nutrients, they won't reach toxic levels in your body, like taking some supplements can cause. This is why one of my main cancer-prevention guidelines is to choose food first and to not take supplements to keep nutrient levels within normal limits. The only time a supplement may be recommended is when a medical-lab draw shows a micronutrient deficiency that you cannot improve with food alone.

That's why it's important to eat a wide variety of colors.

You can easily add a rainbow of fruits and veggies to your diet and reduce cancer risk! You can get started by increasing the amount and variety of plant foods you consume, including fruits, vegetables, grains, beans, lentils, nuts and seeds. There are several reasons why plant foods should be plentiful in a healthy diet:

- Plant foods have fiber; fiber reduces cancer risk.
- Plant foods are low in calorie density, which can help you maintain a healthy weight and help you reduce the risk of the thirteen cancers associated with being overweight and obesity:

  - Breast
  - Colorectal
  - Endometrial
  - Esophageal
  - Gallbladder
  - Kidney
  - Liver

  - Oral
  - Ovarian
  - Pancreatic
  - Prostate
  - Stomach
  - Throat (pharynx and larynx)

- Plant foods are rich in vitamins, minerals and other nutrients that protect cell DNA and repair damaged cells that otherwise would have led to cancer (thank you, plants, for coming to the rescue!).

SEVEN FUN AND SIMPLE WAYS TO EAT A MORE PLANT-FORWARD DIET

1. Add more beans, peas, lentils—whole or mashed—to your meals and snacks. Chickpeas are great in salads. Beans of all kinds work in pasta and other grain-based dishes. Hummus-style dips can be made from any type of legume.

2. Enjoy roasted vegetables (such as eggplant, bell peppers, summer squash, mushrooms, butternut squash, Brussels sprouts and broccoli) as starters, side dishes, salads, baked potato toppings, omelet/scrambled egg additions and flatbread topping options.

3. Make fruit your add-on or main ingredient for your dessert choices. This means you will consume more cancer-protective and immunity-protective properties such as fiber, vitamin C, potassium and phytonutrients. If you want a bit more sweetness or depth of flavor to an all-fruit dessert, you can drizzle honey, sprinkle fragrant spices (cardamom or cinnamon), use yogurt as a dip or top with whipped cream.

4. Add plants into smoothies. Jump-start your day or midday snack with a plant-powered smoothie. Start building from your veggie drawer—veggies like beets, avocados, collard greens and even fresh herbs are fair game for your morning mix-up.

5. Pack some vegetables into your lunch or have them as a snack. Baby carrots, sliced bell peppers or zucchini, broccoli and cauliflower are perfect for snacking on. Make a healthy veggie dip by adding some spices (onion, garlic, dill etc.) to low-fat sour cream or low-fat Greek yogurt, and put some in a small container to eat with the veggies.

6. Try replacing one meat dish once a week. If you are working on reducing meat intake, start small. Try replacing one meal a week with a vegetarian source of protein. For example, try using crumbled tofu to replace ground meat. Add some taco seasoning to the tofu and voilà, you have a delicious and nutrient-dense meat alternative!

7. Stock your fridge and pantry with plant-based foods. If you have plant foods on hand, you are more likely to eat them. Plant foods include fruit and vegetables (fresh, frozen or canned); lentils and beans; nuts and seeds; grains such as rice, oats, bulgur, barley, millet and quinoa and foods made of them, such as breads, pasta and cereal and soy products such as tofu and soy milk.

THE MANY BENEFITS OF WHOLE GRAINS

Diets rich in whole grains protect against cancer, diabetes and heart disease.

Whole grain benefits in detail:

- They break down more slowly in the body: Whole grains contain all three parts of the grain (the bran, germ and endosperm), whereas refined grains are mainly just the endosperm. When all three parts are available in the food you're consuming, your body digests it more slowly. Ultimately, this makes it easier for your body to regulate blood sugars.
- They are high in fiber: High-fiber foods are filling and, therefore, discourage overeating. Plus, when combined with plenty of fluid, they help move food through the digestive system to prevent constipation and reduce risk for colon cancer.
- They provide vitamins and minerals: Whole grains contain important vitamins and minerals, such as B vitamins, magnesium, folate, calcium, potassium, phosphorus, zinc and iron, all of which help to support your brain function and supply day-to-day energy!

Whole grains (starches) are found in many foods, such as potatoes, oats, cereals and breads. Starches are more complex, containing hundreds or even thousands of units of monosaccharides and ultimately take longer for the body to break down. These amazing whole grains, like brown rice, oatmeal and whole-grain breads and cereals, are the way to go.

Unrefined whole grains retain many vital nutrients and are rich in fiber, which helps your digestive system work well and reduces risk for cancer.

> Aim for 30 grams of fiber each day to reduce risk of colon cancer!

Complex carbohydrate foods to include in your diet:

- Whole grain cereals
- Legumes/beans
- Brown rice
- Whole grain breads
- Starchy and non-starchy vegetables

For people who need to avoid gluten, such as those with celiac disease, it's still important to include whole grains. Gluten-free whole grains include amaranth, quinoa, buckwheat, corn, millet, teff, brown rice and wild rice. Many other gluten-free grain products are refined grains that are low in fiber and protective compounds, thus not as well-rounded of a choice for your body.

CHOOSING PROTEIN THAT KEEPS YOU STRONG

Protein is another vital nutrient to make sure you are getting enough of during and after cancer treatment. About 20 percent of the human body is made up of protein. Because your body doesn't store protein, it's important to get enough from your diet each day!

For most adults, a good goal to begin with is 20 to 30 grams of protein at meals and around 10 to 15 grams of protein with snacks. Proteins are the major structural materials for all cells in your body and are responsible for replacing expired and damaged cells whenever your body is growing or repairing itself. How much protein you need depends on several factors, including age, sex, treatment plan, health status and activity level.

FOODS THAT CONTAIN PROTEIN

Protein can be found in both animal and plant-based foods. Some sources of protein are considered better choices than others because of their influence on heart health and cancer-risk factors.

When considering where to focus on protein foods, start with low-fat dairy products, skinless poultry, fish, beans, lentils and soy foods such as tofu and tempeh.

> Nutritious protein options you can begin incorporating during or after cancer treatment:
>
> - **Meat, poultry and eggs:** lean cuts of beef, lamb, goat, pork loin, skinless chicken and turkey, quail and duck and fortified omega-3 eggs
> - **Fish and seafood:** salmon, tuna, cod, shrimp, mackerel, lobster, catfish and crab
> - **Low-fat dairy foods:** yogurt, milk, cheese and cottage cheese
> - **Legumes:** beans, split peas, lentils and soy
> - **Nuts and seeds:** walnuts, almonds, chia seeds, pumpkin seeds, pistachios, cashews and peanuts (whole or crushed)

ANIMAL PROTEIN BENEFITS AND DRAWBACKS

Eating animal protein sources has a wealth of benefits for your health. Moderate amounts in your diet can provide protein, iron, zinc and vitamin B12.

The type of animal protein you pick matters, too! Certain sources like fish have additional health benefits, such as lowering rates of cognitive decline and heart disease. When you prioritize animal protein in your diet, you're also putting yourself in a position to increase your lean muscle mass in combination with weight or resistance training while simultaneously reducing muscle loss that happens as you age.

However, there are some downsides to eating certain types of animal protein. For example, eating more than 18 ounces (510 g) of red meat each week (approximately five 3-ounce servings) can increase cancer risk. Additionally, processed meat has been known to also increase risk of colorectal cancer when eaten in excess. When you eat processed meats daily (like hot dogs and cold cuts), you can increase your risk of colorectal cancer risk by 16 percent!

As with all foods, it's important to make informed choices so you can feed your body what it needs to perform its best and keep you healthy.

Some foods rich in protein may also be high in saturated fat or be considered processed meat. High intakes of saturated fat are not ideal, as these may increase risk for heart disease. There is also strong evidence that processed meats increase risk for cancer—eating it can increase your risk of bowel and stomach cancer. For processed meat, every 50 grams (about one hot dog or two slices of ham) eaten daily raises the risk of colorectal cancer by 16 percent.

As a general rule, limit protein foods that are high in saturated fats or processed meats, such as:

- **Meats and poultry:** chicken-fried steak, fried chicken, organ meats, spare ribs and high-fat meat cuts
- **Fish and shellfish:** breaded and fried options
- **Whole-fat dairy:** whole milk and other whole-fat dairy products
- **Processed meat:** bacon, precooked sausages, hot dogs and lunch meats

PLANT PROTEIN BENEFITS

Plant-based proteins are important because they contain compounds that protect our DNA. Incorporating plant proteins is important for your overall health because they offer many vitamins, minerals, antioxidants, phytonutrients *and* protein (seriously, they're awesome!). Adding more plant protein to your daily, weekly and monthly diet can also help reduce your consumption of red meats and processed meats, which in turn will help minimize the risk of colorectal cancer.

Let's take a look at individual plant proteins you can begin to eat more often starting today!

Soy products (tofu, tempeh, edamame): Soy is the only plant protein that is considered a "complete protein." This means soy contains all the essential amino acids, just like meat does! Tofu is an excellent replacement for meat, and studies show it can help reduce the risk of breast cancer.

Beans (kidney, black, pinto, garbanzo, etc.): Beans are all high in protein; you can pair them with brown rice to make them a complete protein.

Lentils: Lentils contain 18 grams of protein per cooked cup; pair that with rice for more protein. *Note that 1 cup (198 g) of lentils provides about 50 percent of your daily dietary fiber needs.*

Seitan: Seitan is another great and popular protein source; it is made from gluten, which is the main protein in wheat. Seitan will provide about 25 grams of protein per 3½ ounces.

Spelt and teff: Spelt and teff offer 10 to 11 grams of protein per cup. Beyond protein, these grains provide healthy complex carbs, fiber, iron, magnesium, phosphorus, manganese, B vitamins, zinc and selenium, and that's a lot of great cancer prevention properties!

LOWERING CANCER RISK WITH LESS SALT

Stomach, or gastric, cancer is the fifth most common cancer in the world and has few symptoms. Cancer prevention through diet and lifestyle is especially important.

Sodium is an essential mineral that helps your muscles function and controls fluid balances. But too much sodium can increase your risk of stomach cancer. Research has shown that excess salt consumption can actually damage the stomach lining and cause lesions. When left untreated, the lesions can turn cancerous.

> If you are able to cut down on the amount of salt you eat, you can significantly reduce your risk of stomach cancer.

Diets high in sodium can often be a clue that you're eating many foods with added salt that are also highly processed foods, fast foods and processed meats like sausage, hot dogs and bacon. This may mean you're not getting enough vegetables, fruit, legumes and other plant-based foods known to lower the risk for cancer.

The following are examples of salty foods to look out for:

- Any smoked, cured, salted or canned meat, fish or poultry. Some of those items include bacon, cold cuts, hot dogs, sausages, etc.
- Frozen breaded meats and dinners, such as burritos and pizza
- Canned entrees, such as ravioli, spam and chili
- Salted nuts
- Beans canned with added salt

Sodium is typically associated with salt, but the two aren't the same thing. Table salt is a seasoning that contains sodium. One teaspoon of salt contains 2,300 mg of sodium—the sodium content in a serving of food is listed on the label for you to check out.

FIVE SIMPLE WAYS TO REDUCE YOUR SODIUM INTAKE

Try the following hacks to help you reduce your sodium intake:

1. Cook at home. Cooking at home gives you more control over how much salt is in your food. Try salt-free seasonings such as onions, garlic, herbs, spices and vinegar to flavor foods instead of using extra salt.

2. Avoid spice blends that include salt. For example, choose onion powder over onion salt, and go for seasoning mixes that are reduced-, low- or no-sodium options from the supermarket. Additionally, turmeric, the ingredient that makes curry powder yellow, is being studied for anti-inflammatory properties that may help to prevent cancer. Sweet spices like cinnamon, ginger and cloves may also help prevent cell damage.

3. Choose your foods carefully at the grocery store. Whenever possible, choose fresh foods. Processed, prepared and packaged foods are some of the biggest sources of extra sodium to our diets. Remember, check the label for low sodium, no salt added or no sodium on your favorite food items.

4. Check sodium levels in food labels. A good rule of thumb is to try to limit the processed foods that are above 400 mg of sodium per serving to keep to the overall 2,300 mg of sodium per day.

5. Make lower-sodium choices at restaurants. Request that your meal be prepared without salt (this may be more challenging in certain restaurants if their protein sources arrive pre-salted). You can also ask for sauces and salad dressings to be served on the side.

ALL ABOUT DIETARY FAT SOURCES

Fat provides the body with calories for growth, physical activity, hormone production, vitamin transportation and building new cells. We need fat in our diets to keep healthy and strong to feel our best.

We all need to eat a small amount of fat to have a healthy and balanced diet. *The right amount of fat helps our bodies do the following:*

- Stay warm
- Have energy
- Produce hormones that help our bodies function properly
- Have essential fatty acids, such as omega-3 and omega-6, which the body cannot make
- Absorb vitamins A, D and E, which the body can't absorb without the help of fat

There's a lot of misinformation out there about fats, but I need you to understand that you do not need to fear fats after cancer.

During treatment, if you're having difficulty with treatment-related weight loss, eating more higher-fat foods can help you add those needed calories to maintain your weight.

When it comes to dietary fats, there are three types:

- Unsaturated fats
    - Polyunsaturated fats: Have these healthy fats in small amounts and with all meals. They supply omega-3 and omega-6. Your body can't make these important nutrients on its own. Examples of polyunsaturated fats include:
        - *oily fish like kippers, mackerel and salmon; rapeseed oil, sunflower oil and corn oil and walnuts, pine nuts, sesame seeds and sunflower seeds.*
    - Monounsaturated fats: Have these healthy fats in small amounts. They include:
        - *peanut butter, almonds, cashews, hazelnuts, peanuts and pistachios and olive oil, olives and avocados.*

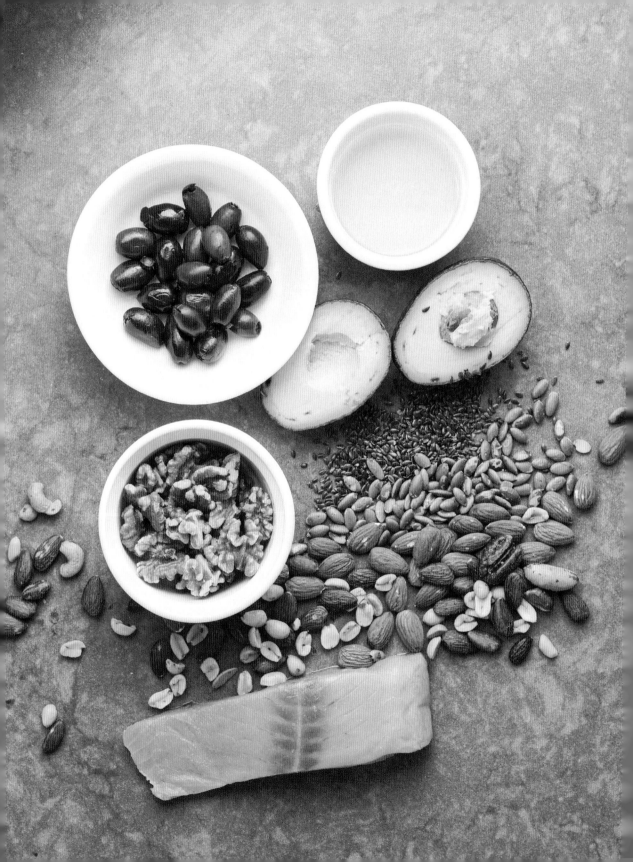

- Saturated fats
  - Reduce how much you eat of these unhealthy fats by swapping some of them for unsaturated fats. Saturated fats include:
    - *processed and fatty meats such as sausages, ham, burgers and bacon; hard cheeses such as Cheddar, whole milk, cream and ice cream and butter, lard, ghee, suet, palm oil and coconut oil.*
- Trans fats
  - Drastically limit how much you eat of these unhealthy fats, including:
    - *fried and take-out foods; snacks such as biscuits, cakes, pies and pastries and hard margarines made with hydrogenated oil.*

BUT WHAT ABOUT CANCER RISK?

Studies show mixed results as to whether saturated fat is responsible for increasing cancer risk. Something we do know is that excess calories that lead to weight gain can increase cancer risk. This is because adipose (fat) tissue can secrete growth hormones that can promote cancer.

In general, people who tend to have a diet high in saturated fat tend to eat calorically dense foods overall, contributing to excess weight gain and thus a higher risk of cancer.

Easy tips to help you reduce unhealthy fats (and increase the healthy ones!):

- Cook with vegetable oils and spreads like olive oil, rapeseed oil and sunflower oil.
- Measure the amount of oil you use with a teaspoon or use a spray bottle.
- Make your sandwich fillers healthier by using spreads made from vegetable oils and nuts. And swap hard cheese and processed meat for oily fish and vegetables like avocado and lettuce.
- Reduce your intake of processed meats like sausages. Choose lean meats (meats with less fat) like lean red meats, skinless chicken, turkey, fish and seafood or plant-based protein like lentils or beans.
- Snack on fruit or unsalted nuts rather than biscuits, cakes and chips.
- Use 1 to 2 percent–fat milk or plant-based milk like almond, soy, oat and cashew milk. Be mindful that plant-based milks (except soy) are lower in protein, so be sure to make up for that with other protein sources.
- Grate your cheese to make it go further in your meal.
- Check the amount of saturated fat per serving on your food labels to help you keep to the recommended daily intake.

THE TRUTH ABOUT SUGAR AND CANCER

Cancer cells require extra energy throughout the entirety of the growth process. These cells can change their energy consumption, unlike with healthy cells. When their healthy neighbor cells break down proteins into amino acid building blocks, the cancer cells absorb these and use them to grow. The cancer cells are able to trick their neighboring healthy cells into supplying them with energy so they can make use of sugars and amino acids from the bloodstream to grow and divide indefinitely.

The most prominent change is the increased tumor glycolysis that leads to increased glucose uptake and utilization. However, it has become obvious that many non-glucose nutrients, like amino acids, lactate, acetate and macro-molecules, can be alternative fuels for cancer cells. This knowledge reveals an unexpected flexibility in which cancer cells uptake nutrients from their external environment to fulfill their necessary energetic needs.

Most people are aware of popular myths like "cancer loves sugar," "cancer thrives off of sugar," or "sugar feeds cancer." However, they are missing three key details:

1. Cancer uses what seems like endless metabolic adaptations to remain nourished using non-glucose nutrients.

2. Cancer is able to adapt and reprogram pathways and metabolites to support metabolism to keep growing regardless of diet (*cancer cannot be controlled with diet or cutting out single foods, like sugar*).

3. Healthy cells still need proper nutrition to withstand and then repair themselves throughout the treatment process.

DO NOT TRY TO STARVE CANCER

Cancer's ability to be flexible and adaptive when it comes to where and how to get fuel has been demonstrated over and again. In fact, cancer cells are intelligent enough that they contain nutrient-sensing pathways, meaning they can survive any nutrient limitations, or starvation, in their environment.

DO NOT try to starve cancer as it WILL NOT WORK!

Your cancer will thrive and your healthy cells will suffer. Always prioritize food intakes to avoid malnutrition and to protect and help repair healthy cells throughout treatment. The more that you take care of your healthy cells, the more they will take care of you. Healthy cells could mean less-severe side effects, fewer missed treatments and fewer instances of reduced-treatment doses.

Which leads us back again to our primary focus: nourishing healthy cells instead of attempting the impossible task of "starving" such adaptable and greedy cancer cells.

ARE SOME CARBS "BAD"?

Are some carbs bad? In short, no. No single food can cause cancer, and no carbs are "bad." In fact, in order to feel more balanced and at ease with foods you love, it's best to not omit any foods and/or declare that any foods are "off-limits," as this can lead to overeating or binging.

Now, with that being said, there are two types of carbohydrate groups: complex and simple. The carbs that are simple are less nutrient dense and are going to be sugary and refined foods. These are typically easy to obtain, come in large portions, taste good and aren't too filling. For instance, sugar is a simple carbohydrate. You may have heard claims like the following about them:

"Sugar feeds cancer."
"Sugar is addictive."
"Sugar is the root of all health issues."
"Sugar is really poison."

These are ridiculous notions about a simple carbohydrate. Phrases like these are why so many survivors are unsure if they should have sugar and worry it'll either cause cancer or bring it back quickly. This is not true at all.

Cancer is not caused by sugar. If you eat sugar, your cancer will not grow more quickly, just as if you were to omit it, cancer would not grow more slowly. You can choose to omit high-sugar, low-nutrition simple carbohydrates, such as soda and candy. However, that's not realistic or necessary, as most people enjoy a soda at times, dessert, a sweet snack, birthday cake, an ice cream date and so on.

As I stated previously, I am not advocating a high-sugar diet at all, but you can still make a lot of room for a diet filled with all carbohydrates and have a part of that allowance include those sugary foods you love and want to enjoy throughout life, as most people do.

Simple carbs are also found in many nutritious foods, such as fruits, vegetables and dairy products, which provide a range of essential nutrients that support our gut health, immune system and cognitive functioning and reduce cancer risk. Fresh fruits, for example, contain simple carbs but also have vitamins, antioxidants and fiber.

The bottom line: Simple carbohydrates are very safe after cancer. Choose more fruit, whole grains and lean dairy choices (1 to 2 percent fat) more often and choose sodas, juices and table sugars less often.

THE ONLY TWO THINGS TO REMOVE FROM YOUR DIET TO REDUCE CANCER RISK

Alcohol and processed meats are the only beverage and dietary items for which there is significant evidence to show they do increase risk of cancer. These are the only two things that the World Cancer Research Fund recommends you eliminate after cancer. They are simply not part of a cancer-prevention lifestyle.

What are processed meats and what do they have to do with cancer risk?

Processed meat is any meat (including fish) preserved by using smoking, curing, fermentation, salting and/or the addition of chemical preservatives. Examples of processed meats include but are not limited to the following:

- Bacon
- Beef jerky
- Deli meats and cold cuts
- Ham
- Hot dogs

- Pancetta
- Pepperoni
- Salami
- Sausage

Why is processed meat something we should omit or limit? Processed meat has repeatedly been shown to increase the risk of certain cancers, such as stomach and colorectal cancers. We also know processed meats can harm cardiovascular health. A report from the AICR (American Institute for Cancer Research), *Diet, Nutrition, Physical Activity, and Cancer: A Global Perspective*, found that regularly eating even small amounts of cold cuts and other processed meats can increase the risk of colorectal cancer.

Every 50 grams of processed meat eaten daily (about two slices of deli meat) could increase the risk of colon cancer by 16 percent.

Why does processed meat increase cancer risk? It's not yet clear exactly why processed meats increase risk for colorectal cancer. Researchers are currently exploring a few possible mechanisms, including the following:

- Nitrates/nitrites: These substances are added to processed meats to preserve color and prevent spoilage. In lab studies, they form cancer-causing compounds called carcinogens.

- Smoking: Smoked meats contain PAHs (polycyclic aromatic hydrocarbons), substances that are formed at high heat and considered carcinogenic.

- Cooking at high temperatures: Meats cooked at high temperatures can also contain PAHs and HCAs (heterocyclic amines), which can damage DNA.

- Heme iron: The heme iron found in red meat may damage the lining of the colon.

WORKING TOWARD AN ALCOHOL-FREE LIFESTYLE

Alcohol use is the third-leading modifiable factor that increases cancer risk, after cigarette smoking and excess body weight. Research has found that choosing even less than one drink per day—of any kind of alcohol—can help reduce your overall cancer risk.

- ALL alcohol increases cancer risk.
- Alcohol is metabolized into acetaldehyde, which is a carcinogen; this damages our DNA.
- Alcohol robs the body of vitamins, specifically B vitamins and vitamin D.
- Alcohol molecules can help bring other cancer-causing molecules into cells.
- Omit alcohol to reduce cancer risk, or work on reducing alcohol intake.

The following cancers are associated with alcohol intake:

- Breast
- Colon
- Colorectal
- Esophageal
- Liver
- Oral
- Stomach
- Throat (pharynx and larynx)

Skip drinking wine for the "benefits."

There are no benefits to alcohol. Wine being "heart healthy" is not supported by any solid data.

There's a debate about whether or not resveratrol is truly cardioprotective. In addition, there is debate about the amount of resveratrol you would need to ingest to get a protective effect. To get the equivalent of the amount of resveratrol that has been reported to be protective would probably mean ingesting an excess of wine.

Instead, eat whole grapes to reduce cancer risk! Resveratrol and a wide variety of phytocompounds found in grapes are likely to help the fruit play a role in the diet to reduce cancer risk.

DOES THE TYPE OF ALCOHOL MATTER?

Ethanol is the type of alcohol found in alcoholic drinks. While different alcoholic drinks contain different amounts of ethanol, a general, standard-sized drink of any type of alcohol has about the same amount of ethanol per serving. If the size of the drink increases, so does the amount of ethanol.

Based on the recent research, the type of alcohol that's being consumed is not as important as the amount that a person is drinking over time. The risk according to the research is the consumption of ethanol, not the other things in the drink.

For cancer prevention, the recommendation of alcohol consumption is zero drinks per day. It does not matter the type of alcoholic drink, as the cancer risk comes from ethanol. Whether it is wine, beer, spirits or other alcoholic beverages we drink, they are classified as a type called ethyl alcohol, or ethanol.

When it is too hard to remove alcohol completely, you can try these hacks:

- Avoid asking for a double.
- Alternate alcoholic and non-alcoholic drinks.
- Keep some days alcohol-free each week.
- Enjoy low- or no-alcohol alternative drinks (such as non-alcoholic beer).
- Be aware that restaurants and bars often serve larger than standard-sized alcoholic drinks.
- Sip slowly, as you'll be less likely to finish the drink quickly and overconsume.
- Order smaller sizes.

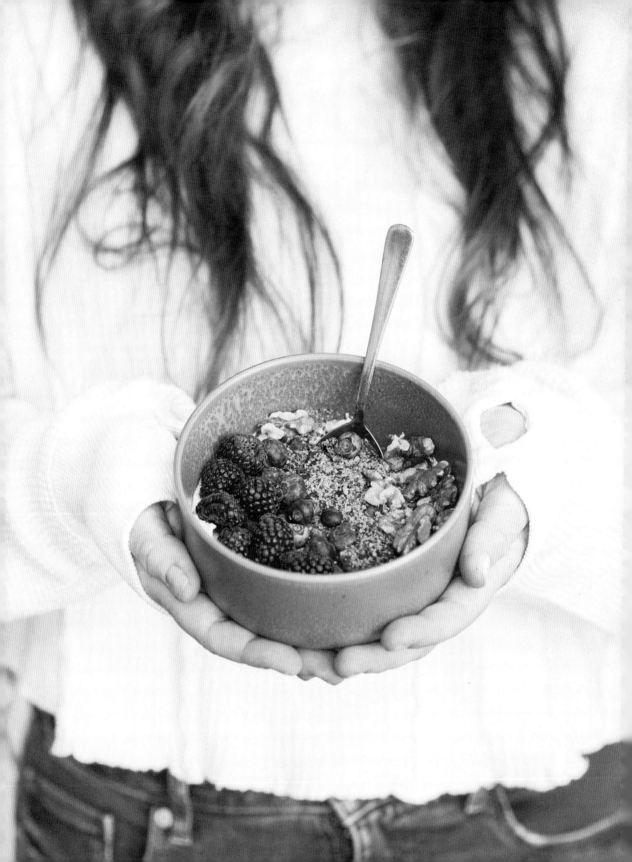

SIMPLE,
NUTRITIOUS
Breakfasts

Breakfast is an exciting and very important meal of the day and can easily be filled with cancer-prevention ingredients you will love! I have come up with breakfast ideas that are filled with variety and flavor and are simple! Pour a cup of coffee (or tea, as both are safe and should be a part of a cancer-prevention lifestyle!), and let's get cooking! From recipes full of tasty berries, crunch and healthy fats from seeds and nuts, to fancy-enough-for-holiday breakfast, to just plain old simple and fiber-filled easy breakfast ideas before you head off to work, I've got you covered! Let's dive in!

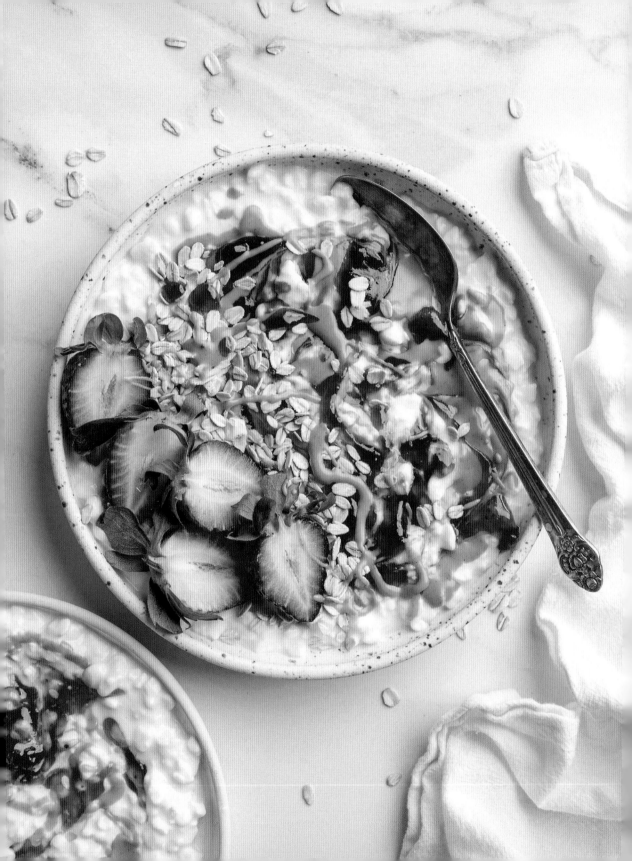

COTTAGE CHEESE BOWLS

Yield: 1 serving per each bowl

PEANUT BUTTER & JELLY BOWL

½ cup (113 g) 2% cottage cheese

¼ cup (23 g) rolled oats

1 tbsp (20 g) jam (any flavor)

1 tbsp (16 g) smooth peanut butter

THE SAVORY BOWL

½ cup (113 g) 2% cottage cheese

1 large hard-boiled egg

6 grape tomatoes, halved

6 slices cucumber, skin on or off, as you prefer

Dash of freshly cracked black pepper

APPLE-CINNAMON BOWL

½ cup (113 g) 2% cottage cheese

½ apple, chopped

1 tbsp (14 g) chopped walnuts

1 tbsp (15 ml) maple syrup

Dash of cinnamon

Ready for some quick, sweet and savory breakfast bowls that are also higher in protein? Yum! Cottage cheese is a low-calorie cheese with a mild flavor. Its popularity has grown in the last few decades, and it's often recommended as part of a healthy diet. One cup (226 g) of cottage cheese has a whopping 28 grams of protein! It's also packed with many nutrients, such as B vitamins, calcium, phosphorus and selenium. Colon cancer risk is reduced when consuming dairy products, which is even more reason to enjoy this versatile food!

For each of the three cottage cheese bowls, add the cottage cheese first, then place the other ingredients on top. You can then enjoy each bowl immediately or refrigerate in an airtight container for up to 4 days.

TOAST WITH SUNFLOWER SEED BUTTER AND PEACHES

Yield: 1 serving

1 medium peach
2 slices whole wheat bread
2 oz (57 g) sunflower seed butter
1 oz (28 g) pumpkin seeds

One medium peach is only 40 calories, has 2 grams of fiber, 285 mg of potassium and a fair amount of vitamin A. This yummy treat also uses whole grain bread, which is a good choice to include in a diet that reduces cancer risk. Whole grains provide fiber, vitamins, minerals and other nutrients. A treat when sliced into fruit or green salads, peaches are prime for pies, too.

Cut the peach into eight slices. Toast the bread and lay each slice on a plate. Spread evenly with 1 ounce (28 g) of sunflower seed butter on each slice. Top the sunflower seed butter with peach slices by laying them in an even layer. Sprinkle the pumpkin seeds on top.

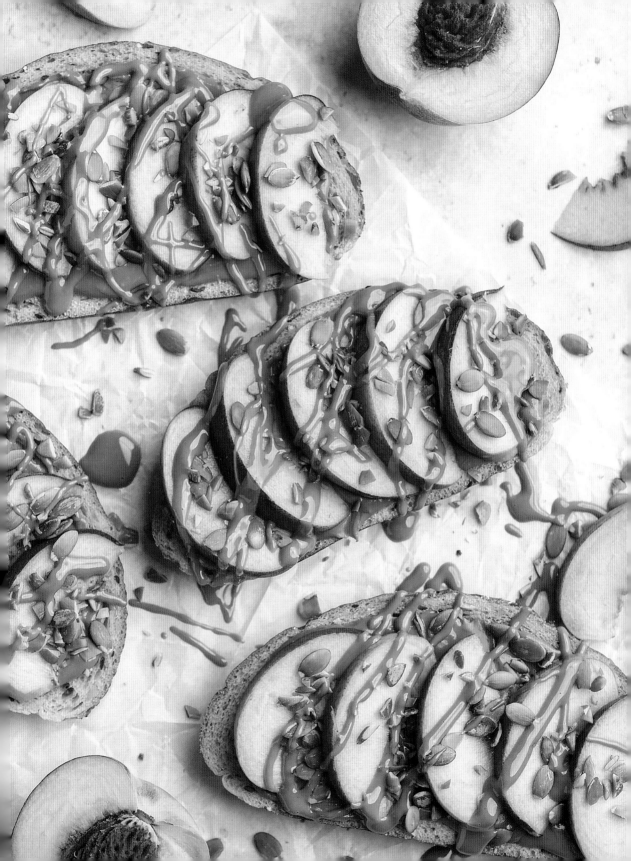

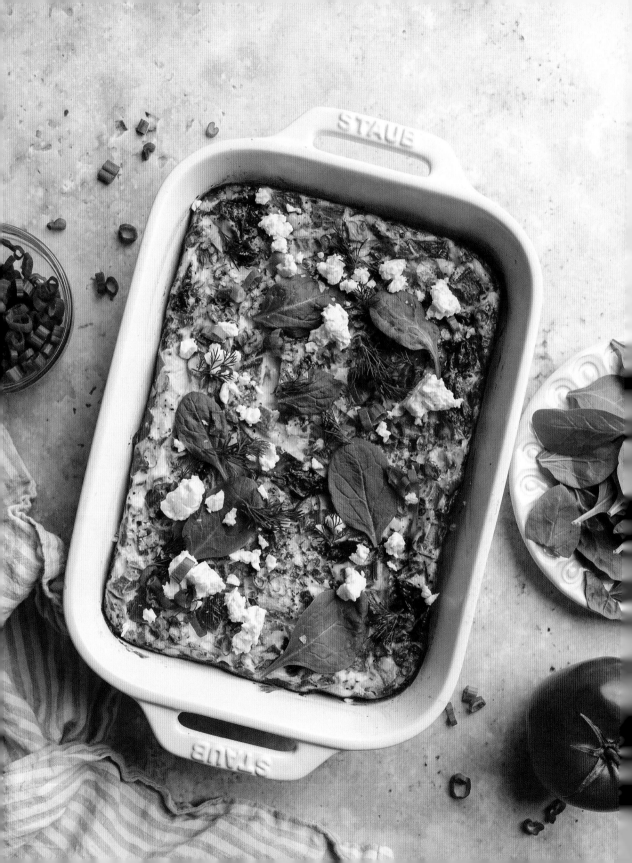

TOMATO, SPINACH AND FETA BREAKFAST CASSEROLE

Yield: 12 servings

Olive oil spray
1 tsp olive oil
3 shallots, chopped
1 (6-oz [23-g]) bag baby spinach
10 large eggs, plus 10 egg whites, beaten
2½ cups (600 ml) milk of your choice
1½ cups (225 g) feta cheese, crumbled
3 scallions, chopped
3 plum tomatoes, seeded and diced
Black pepper, to taste

This easy breakfast casserole is made with eggs, spinach, tomatoes and feta cheese and only takes a few minutes to whip up. You can make it ahead of time, so it's the perfect breakfast casserole for holiday mornings or any day! The great thing about this recipe is how adaptable it is! And because this dish is deep, you can pack tons more ingredients in it! Here are some ideas to make an epic breakfast casserole:

- Add more veggies! Bell peppers, zucchini and mushrooms would all be great options.

- Try different cheese options. Swap out the feta cheese for ricotta, Parmesan, Swiss or Cheddar.

- Add some herbs. Chopped dill, parsley or chives would make a great addition.

Preheat the oven to 350°F (180°C). Spray a 9 x 13–inch (23 x 33–cm) glass baking dish with olive oil spray.

Heat a large skillet over medium heat. Add the olive oil and shallots and cook until soft, 6 to 8 minutes. Add the spinach and cook until wilted. Remove from the heat.

In a large bowl, whisk the eggs and egg whites, milk, feta, scallions, tomatoes and black pepper. Mix in the spinach and shallots and pour the mixture into the prepared dish. Bake until the center is solid and cooked through, about 1 hour and 20 minutes.

GREEK YOGURT POWER BOWL WITH BERRIES AND NUTS

Yield: 1 serving

1 cup (240 ml) plain 2% Greek yogurt

2 tbsp (24 g) whole blueberries

2 tbsp (16 g) whole raspberries

2 tbsp (28 g) walnuts, whole or chopped

2 tbsp (20 g) whole or ground seed blend or seed of choice (I use a hemp-chia-flax blend)

This Greek yogurt recipe combines seeds of your choice, berries and walnuts, which all contain nutrients to reduce inflammation and cancer risk and help improve digestion. If you want, you can add even more ingredients to this fun bowl. Think seasonal fruits, dried fruits, nuts and honey. Let's eat breakfast like cancer-prevention experts with great taste!

Pour the Greek yogurt into a medium-sized bowl, and add the fruits, walnuts and seed blend.

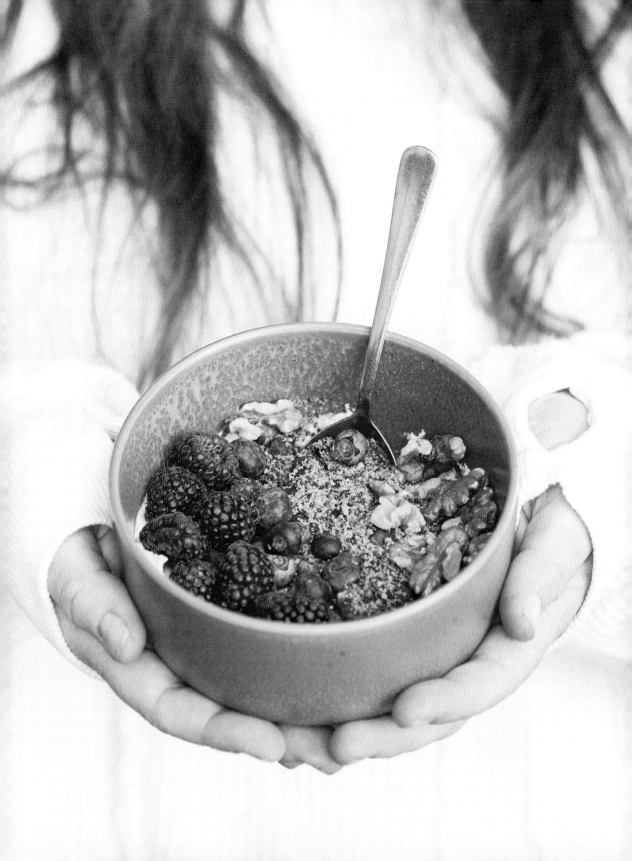

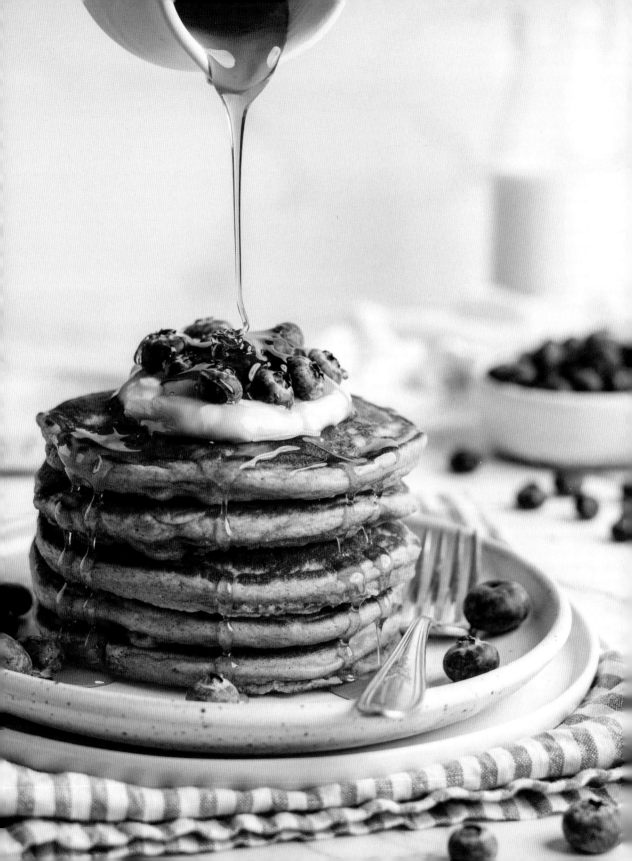

BEST BLUEBERRY PROTEIN PANCAKES

Yield: 4 servings (3 pancakes per serving)

1½ cups (180 g) whole wheat flour

½ cup (48 g) protein powder of your choosing

1½ tsp (7 g) baking powder

½ tsp cinnamon

3 eggs

⅔ cup (160 ml) milk of your choice

Splash of vanilla extract

1 cup (148 g) blueberries

Greek yogurt, to taste

Maple syrup, for drizzling

Blueberries are protective against cancer! They contain a wide range of nutrients, including dietary fiber, vitamin C, flavonols, flavones, tannins and phenolic acids. Several studies found that blueberries can increase antioxidant activity in the blood and scavenge free radicals! This is important for cancer survivors, as it can help prevent further DNA damage.

Whisk together the whole wheat flour, protein powder, baking powder and cinnamon and set aside. In a separate bowl, beat together the eggs and milk. Now you are ready to add a splash of vanilla for a teeny boost of flavor. Pour the egg and milk mixture into the flour mixture, and stir to combine. Fold in the blueberries.

Heat a skillet over medium-low heat and spray it with cooking spray. Drop about a ¼ cup (59 ml) of batter onto the skillet, and cook for 2 to 3 minutes on each side. Repeat with the rest of your batter. Serve the pancakes warm with a dollop of Greek yogurt and maple syrup to taste on each stack of three pancakes.

CORNMEAL BISCUITS WITH STRAWBERRY JAM

Yield: 6 servings

2 cups (332 g) strawberries, trimmed and quartered

2 tbsp (30 ml) maple syrup

½ tsp lemon juice

1½ cups (180 g) whole wheat flour

½ cup (61 g) cornmeal

2 tsp (9 g) baking powder

⅓ cup (75 g) grated butter

⅔ cup (160 ml) buttermilk

Cornmeal and strawberries help reduce cancer risk! Cornmeal is a whole grain, which has been found to reduce colorectal cancer risk. Cornmeal and strawberries contain fiber, phytochemicals, phenolic acids, lignans, B vitamins and minerals. Strawberries support our antioxidant and anti-inflammatory defenses.

Add the strawberries and maple syrup to a saucepan over medium heat. Stir until the mixture begins to bubble. Reduce the heat to low, and let simmer for 10 to 15 minutes, or until the jam begins to thicken. Remove from the heat, add the lemon juice and let the mixture cool down.

Meanwhile, preheat the oven to 400°F (205°C) and line a baking sheet with parchment paper. Mix together the flour, cornmeal and baking powder in a bowl. Add the grated butter, and combine the contents with a fork. Add the buttermilk and keep mixing just until the dough forms.

Transfer the dough to a lightly floured surface. Roll out the dough gently to a ½-inch (1.3-cm) thickness. Use a 2½-inch (6-cm) round cutter and cut the dough into biscuits. Place the biscuits onto the prepared baking sheet. Bake for 12 to 14 minutes, or until lightly golden brown. Serve with the cooked strawberry jam.

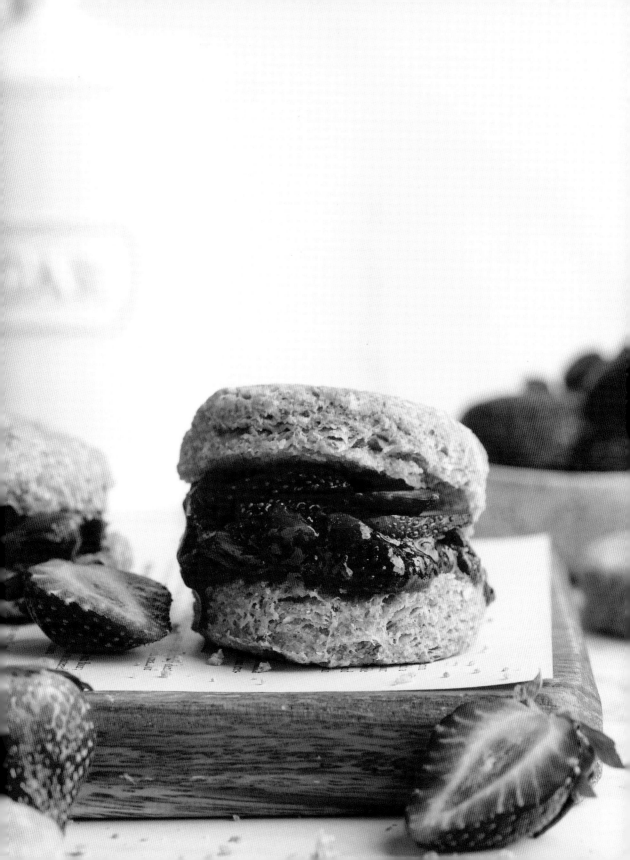

SUPER NUT AND SEED GRANOLA

Yield: 12 servings

This easy nut and seed granola recipe is gluten-free and sweetened with a bit of pure maple syrup. Truly a super granola thanks to the healthy fats, iron-boosting ingredients and additional nutrients from flax! This particular nut and seed granola is made with four different kinds of nuts, pumpkin seeds and hempseeds and is naturally sweetened with maple syrup. I created it specifically for anyone who needs an extra boost of iron in their diet or for those who love to refuel with granola after a workout or cancer treatment. It's truly a granola you can feel good about eating.

DRY INGREDIENTS

1 cup (90 g) rolled oats

¼ cup (30 g) whole wheat flour

2 tbsp (20 g) ground flaxseed

2 tsp (6 g) ground cinnamon

¾ cup (109 g) raw cashews

¾ cup (82 g) raw sliced pecans

½ cup (59 g) raw walnuts

½ cup (69 g) raw pumpkin seeds

½ cup (54 g) raw sliced almonds

½ cup (120 g) hempseeds/hearts

1 cup (120 g) unsweetened coconut flakes (not shredded coconut)

WET INGREDIENTS

¼ cup (60 ml) olive oil

¼ cup (60 ml) maple syrup

1 tsp vanilla extract

Preheat the oven to 300°F (150°C). Line a large baking sheet with parchment paper. In a large bowl, stir together the oats, flour, flaxseed, cinnamon, cashews, pecans, walnuts, pumpkin seeds, sliced almonds, hempseeds and coconut flakes. Set aside.

Next, combine the olive oil, maple syrup and vanilla, then pour it over the dry ingredients and mix well until the oats are completely coated. Then spread the granola on the baking sheet in an even layer, and press down using a spatula (we're going to bake it like it's one big cookie!). Bake for 35 to 40 minutes, until golden brown and fragrant.

Once done, remove the pan from the oven, and allow the granola to cool on the baking sheet for 10 to 15 minutes before you break it into large clumps.

Transfer it to an airtight container or large Mason jar. Store on the counter. It's best used within 7 to 10 days.

GOLDEN COCONUT-APPLE OATMEAL

Yield: 1 serving

¾ cup (180 ml) water or milk, plus more as needed

¼ cup (23 g) rolled oats

1 tbsp (10 g) ground flaxseed

½ medium apple, diced

1 tsp unsweetened shredded coconut

1 tsp ground turmeric

½ tsp each of ground ginger, cinnamon and cardamom

Dash of black pepper

Coconut or almond milk, as needed

Walnuts, almonds or cashews, chopped banana and/or mango, almond butter and/or cacao nibs, as desired for topping (optional)

This Golden Coconut-Apple Oatmeal is inspired by golden milk, the popular, creamy drink made with anti-inflammatory turmeric spice! These oats are made with beautiful warming, sweet and savory spices—ginger, cinnamon, cardamom and turmeric—and simmered with flax, apple (also an amazing breast-cancer-risk-reducing food!) and coconut for a filling, satisfying and healthy breakfast.

To enhance the absorption of curcumin, the active ingredient found in turmeric, I added some black pepper. If you're missing one of the spices, that's okay. Just turmeric and either cinnamon or ginger is delicious; cardamom is just a bonus. If you have them all, go for it!

Enjoy as is or top with mango, banana, nuts or cacao nibs and a drizzle of coconut or almond milk.

Bring the water to a boil in a small saucepan, then add all the ingredients and reduce to a light simmer. Add a bit more water or milk if the mixture seems too thick. Cook for 5 minutes, stirring often, then remove from the heat and let sit for a few minutes before transferring to a bowl and adding any desired toppings.

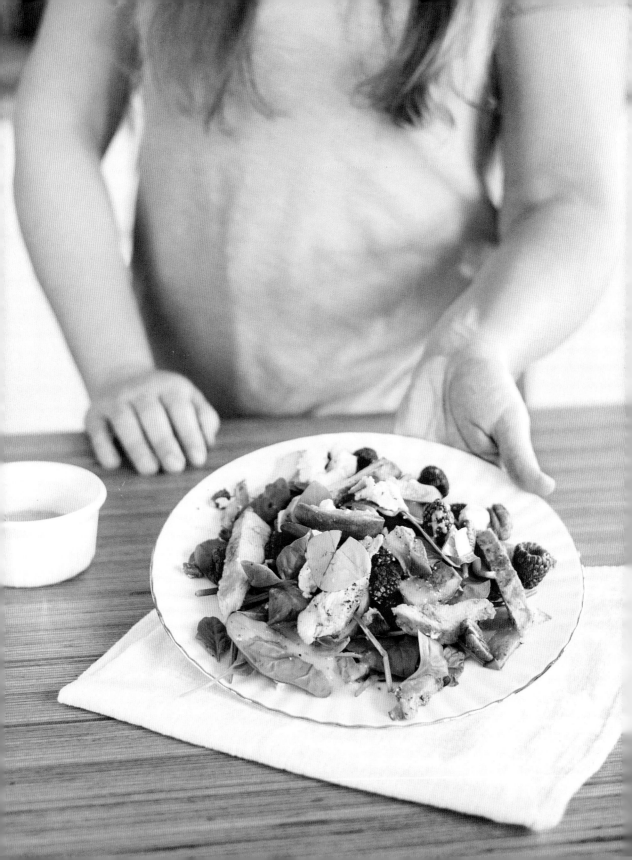

FRESH AND FUN
Lunches

For many, the question "What's for lunch?" comes up more often than not! Most days, people will find themselves staring into the fridge as the clock ticks until their next meeting, hoping lunch will magically present itself (and it never does! ugh!), so snacks become the all-day eats, which do not leave you feeling satisfied. Let's change that! Here are some of my favorite cancer-preventing, easy and fast lunches. Whether it's a big veggie-packed salad recipe you crave; a cold, crisp sandwich; a glorious clean-out-the-fridge grain bowl or something else entirely that you can't quite put your finger on, but you know you want it to be delicious and support your cancer-prevention lifestyle, I know you'll find what you're looking for among these recipes!

Fun lunches? Simple and quick lunches? Ones that also reduce cancer risk? Yup, that is what you will find in this nutrient-packed chapter. Let's do this!

THREE EASY LUNCH FORMULAS THAT DO NOT USE PROCESSED MEATS:

1. Grain bowl: grain + protein + veg + fat/dressing

    - *Whole wheat fusilli + canned tuna + cherry tomatoes, cucumber and onion + olives + lemon-olive oil dressing*
    - *Quinoa + chopped roasted chicken + salad greens + shaved Parmesan + balsamic-olive oil vinaigrette*
    - *Brown rice + crispy baked tofu + sautéed bok choy + crushed peanuts + miso dressing*

2. Soup combo: soup/stew + bread

    - *Turkey-black bean chili + cornbread*
    - *Chickpea stew + drizzle of olive oil + whole wheat sourdough bread*
    - *Chicken taco soup + avocado + whole grain tortilla chips*

3. Sandwich: bread + fat/sauce + protein + veg

    - *Whole wheat everything bagel + hot sauce + avocado + fried eggs (fried in 1 tsp olive oil or cooking spray) + spinach*
    - *Whole wheat sourdough + pesto + sliced roasted chicken + tomato slices and arugula*
    - *Whole wheat pita pockets + tahini or yogurt sauce + baked falafels + tomato, cucumber and onion*

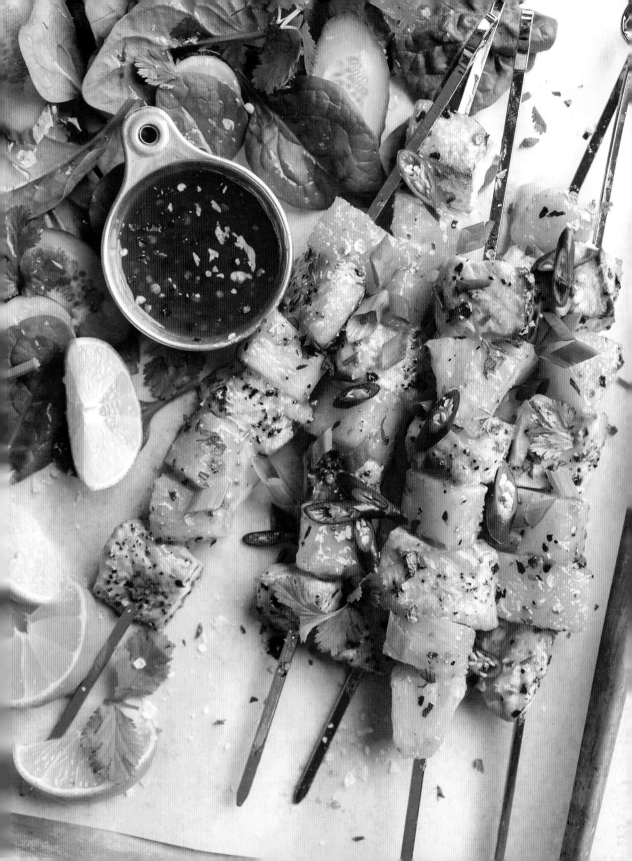

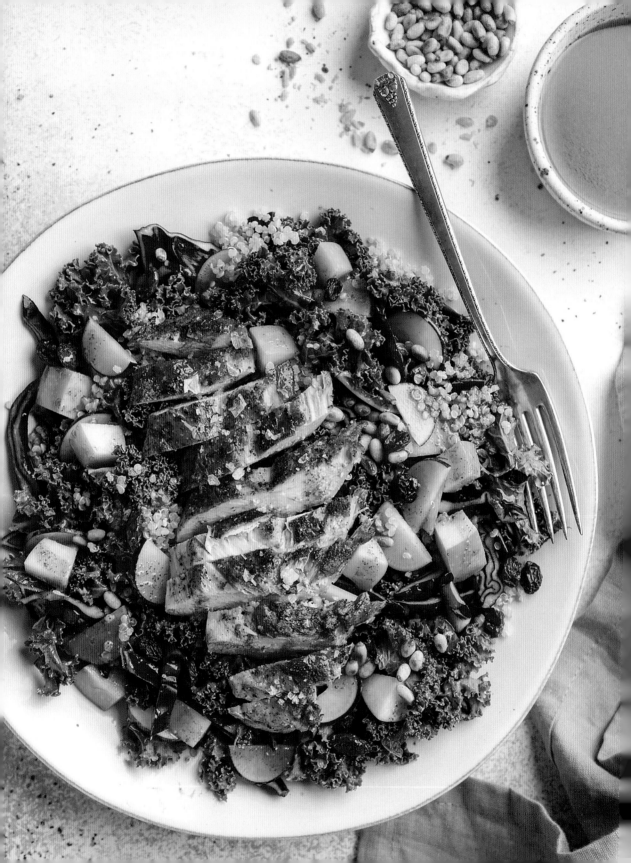

GRILLED CHICKEN, APPLE AND QUINOA SALAD WITH CUMIN VINAIGRETTE

Yield: 4 servings

CHICKEN

16 oz (453 g) skinless chicken breast filets

Pepper, to taste

¼ cup (60 ml) apple cider vinegar

QUINOA

¾ cup (128 g) quinoa

1½ cup (360 ml) water

¼ cup (45 g) raisins

The vitamin C in apples acts as an antioxidant to support immune function and fight cancer cell growth. In addition to preventing tumors, apples also support cancer recovery! In fact, greater consumption of apples specifically was associated with a lower risk of estrogen receptor negative cells (ER-). Here are the essential elements contained in apples: dietary fiber, flavonols and triterpenoid compounds (in the peel).

To prepare the chicken, season the filets generously on both sides with pepper. Place them in a dish and pour the vinegar over them. Refrigerate for about 30 minutes.

While the chicken is marinating, cook the quinoa. Combine the quinoa and water in a saucepan and bring to a boil over high heat. Reduce the heat to low, cover and simmer for about 15 minutes, until the grains are tender and most of the water has been absorbed. Transfer to a large bowl and stir in the raisins.

Preheat the oven to 400°F (205°C). Heat a lightly oiled pan to medium-high heat (you can also use an oven-safe skillet). Remove the chicken from the marinade, discarding the marinade, and pan-fry until browned, about 3 minutes per side. Transfer the chicken to the oven. If you are using an oven-safe skillet or grill pan, you can transfer the whole thing to the oven. Otherwise, place the chicken in a baking dish. Bake for about 15 minutes, until the chicken is cooked through. Remove the chicken from the oven, transfer to a cutting board and let it rest for 10 minutes. Slice into ⅛-inch (3-mm)- thick pieces.

(continued)

GRILLED CHICKEN, APPLE AND QUINOA SALAD WITH CUMIN VINAIGRETTE (CONT.)

VINAIGRETTE

¼ cup (60 ml) apple cider vinegar

1 tbsp (15 ml) Dijon mustard

1 tbsp (15 ml) honey

1 tsp ground cumin

1 tsp paprika

¼ tsp cayenne

⅓ cup (80 ml) olive oil

SALAD

4 radishes, trimmed, halved and thinly sliced

½ bunch kale, julienned

¼ head red cabbage, julienned

1 Granny Smith apple, unpeeled and diced small

GARNISH

2 tbsp (15 g) toasted pine nuts

While the chicken is cooking, make the vinaigrette and the salad. To make the vinaigrette, whisk the vinegar, mustard, honey, cumin, paprika and cayenne in a small bowl, and let it sit for about 5 minutes. Stir in the olive oil.

To make the salad, add the radishes, kale, cabbage and apple to the quinoa and mix well. Add the dressing and toss until well combined. Serve the salad in individual serving bowls, and top with the chicken strips.

Garnish with the pine nuts and serve immediately.

CHICKEN AND STRAWBERRY SPINACH SALAD

Yield : 4 servings

DRESSING

½ cup (120 ml) extra virgin olive oil

2 tbsp (30 ml) apple cider vinegar

2 tbsp (30 ml) fresh lemon juice

1 tbsp (9 g) poppy seeds

½ tsp Dijon mustard

¼ tsp freshly ground black pepper

1 tsp kosher salt

2 chicken breasts, bone-in, skin on

1 tbsp (15 ml) extra virgin olive oil

¼ tsp freshly ground black pepper

Make the most of strawberry season with this light, flavorful Chicken and Strawberry Spinach Salad! Top fresh baby spinach with roasted chicken, strawberries, goat cheese, almonds and a homemade poppy seed dressing. It'll leave you full and savoring a taste that is so amazing!

Spinach contains beta-carotene, vitamin C and fiber along with potential cancer-protective phytochemicals that make it a nutritional powerhouse. What's in spinach that matters? Carotenoids, flavonols, vitamin C, dietary fiber, folate and lignans.

To make the salad dressing, simply combine all the ingredients together in a Mason jar, seal tightly, then shake until well blended. Alternatively, you could place the dressing ingredients in a large measuring cup or mixing bowl and whisk to combine.

To roast the chicken: Preheat the oven to 450°F (230°C). Pat the chicken breasts lightly on all sides with a paper towel, then place the breasts on a parchment-lined baking sheet. Drizzle with the olive oil, then sprinkle with the black pepper. Roast for 45 minutes, or until the skin is crispy and the chicken registers an internal temperature of 165°F (74°C). Allow the chicken to rest for 5 to 10 minutes before carving.

(continued)

CHICKEN AND STRAWBERRY SPINACH SALAD (CONT.)

SALAD

⅔ cup (19 g) fresh baby spinach

1 cup (166 g) strawberries, hulled and quartered

¼ cup (56 g) goat cheese

¼ cup (18 g) sliced almonds

Next, assemble the strawberry salad. Place the baby spinach in a large serving bowl, then add the strawberries, goat cheese and sliced almonds.

Slice the chicken. Use a sharp knife to remove the breast meat from the bone. Place the boneless breast on a cutting board, then slice them into strips about ½-inch (1.3-cm) thick, being careful not to rip the skin. Add the chicken to the salad.

Drizzle as much of the dressing on top as you like, then toss and serve immediately with extra dressing on the side, as desired.

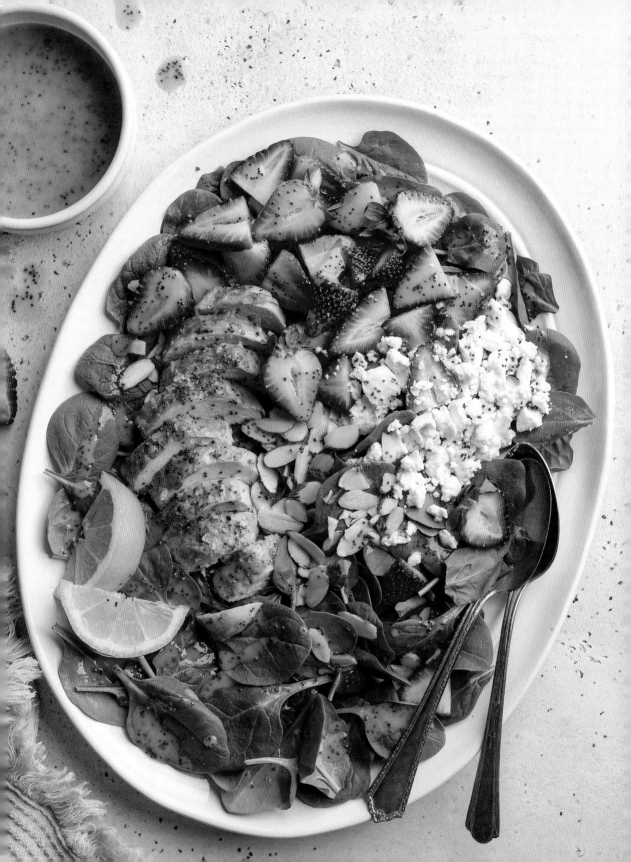

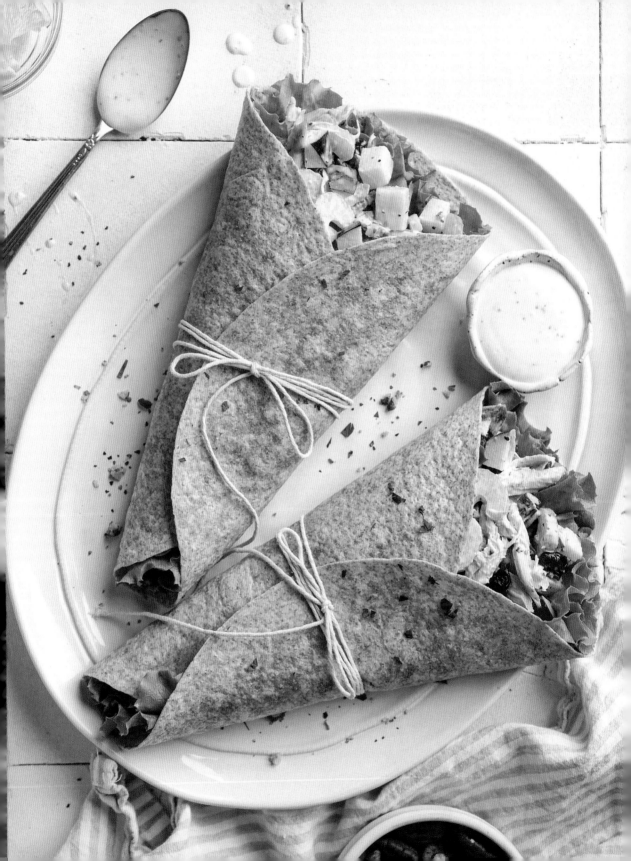

CHICKEN AND CRANBERRY-APPLE WRAP

Yield : 2 servings

3 cups (420 g) precooked chicken, shredded

1 cup (125 g) diced apple

½ cup (55 g) pecans, chopped

⅓ cup (40 g) dried cranberries

2 ribs celery, diced

4 oz (118 ml) mayonnaise

¼ cup (60 ml) plain Greek yogurt

1 tbsp (15 ml) lemon juice

Dash of salt

Dash of black pepper

4 leaves of green leaf lettuce

4 large whole wheat tortillas

These creamy chicken and cranberry-apple salad wraps are the perfect solution for lunch! Filled with shredded chicken, crisp apples and juicy dried cranberries, these wraps have it all! The cancer-protective potential of cranberries comes primarily from a package of phenolic compounds. Balance the fresh cranberries' tartness by mixing them with other fruits, such as oranges and pears, for a relish or salsa.

Combine the shredded chicken, apple, pecans, dried cranberries and ribs of celery in a large bowl.

In a separate, small bowl, combine the mayonnaise, Greek yogurt, lemon juice, salt and pepper. Whisk to combine. Pour the dressing into the chicken mixture and fold until evenly combined.

Place the green leaf lettuce on top of a tortilla, and add a cup (100 g) of chicken mixture on top. Roll up the tortilla, and cut it in half.

PINEAPPLE SALMON SKEWERS

Yield: 4 servings

SALMON

1 lb (450 g) salmon, cut into cubes

Ground pepper, to taste

2½ cups (413 g) cubed pineapple

MARINADE

1½ oz (44 ml) extra virgin olive oil

1½ oz (42 ml) sweet chili sauce

2 cloves garlic, crushed

4 tsp (8 g) freshly grated ginger

⅓ oz (8 ml) sesame oil

1 tsp crushed chili flakes

Salt, to taste

GARNISH

Lime juice, for drizzling

Toasted sesame seeds, as desired

Thinly sliced raw onions, as desired

Salmon is a great choice of protein! It's packed with omega-3s, which support healthy brain function and can combat brain fog, as well as protein, which is extremely important for your healthy cells' repair and growth. To reduce red meat consumption you can also use this salmon steak recipe to replace a beefsteak you might have had otherwise.

Preheat the oven to 325°F (160°C). Season the salmon with pepper. Set aside for 5 minutes while you prepare the marinade.

In a medium bowl, combine the olive oil, chili sauce, garlic, ginger, sesame oil and chili flakes, and season with salt. Whisk until combined. Thread the salmon with the pineapple onto the skewers, alternating until all are used, then brush the skewers with the marinade.

Line a baking tray or sheet pan with parchment paper, and arrange the skewers. Place the tray in the middle rack of the oven. Bake for 12 minutes. Check for doneness using a fork to push through the flesh. The salmon should still be pink but should flake easily. Drizzle with lime juice, and garnish with sesame seeds and onions.

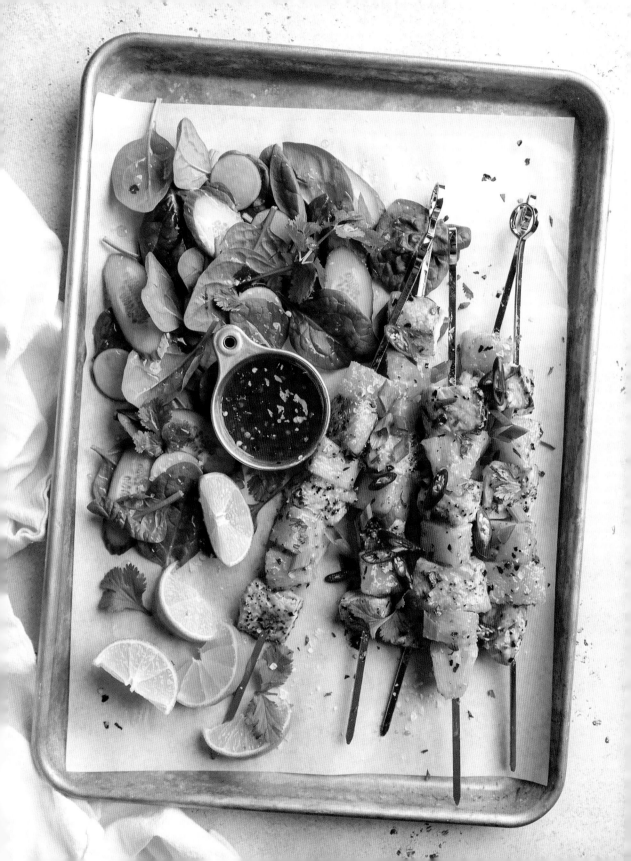

HIGH-PROTEIN LUNCH BOX

Yield : 5 servings

PROTEIN SNACK PACKS

11 oz (305 g) hummus

1⅓ cups (180 g) low-sodium mixed nuts

2¾ cups (340 g) precooked chicken, sliced

1 cup (226 g) Cheddar cheese, chopped into cubes

2½ cups (373 g) cherry tomatoes

1½ cups (95 g) sugar snap peas

1 large English cucumber, sliced

5 eggs, hard-boiled

These high-protein lunch boxes are filled with hard-boiled eggs, almonds, hummus and crunchy veggies. An easy and delicious lunchtime meal-prep solution perfect for any protein lover, these fantastic, little protein snack packs are perfect for school lunches, post-workout snacks or picnics in the park.

Fill five mini plastic or glass cups with lids with hummus and seal (each will hold approximately 2 ounces [59 ml]). Fill five more mini cups with lids with your favorite type of low-sodium nut or nut mix and secure with the lid. Set aside.

Divide the remaining ingredients—the chicken, cheese, cherry tomatoes, sugar snap peas, English cucumber and eggs— among five single-compartment containers. Add one cup filled with hummus and one filled with nuts to each container. Seal and store in the refrigerator for up to 5 days.

THE ULTIMATE CHICKEN AND GRILLED-PEAR SPINACH SALAD

This simple salad recipe is filled with juicy pears, raspberries, goat cheese, pecans and grilled chicken and drizzled with a honey mustard dressing. It's an easy and healthy lunch idea you're going to love! Why do I love you using pecans as much as you can? Pecans contain a high amount of healthy mono- and polyunsaturated fats, which have been suggested to reduce the risk of many types of cancer.

Yield: 2 servings

Preheat a 12-inch (30-cm) grill pan over medium-high heat. Season the chicken with pepper on both sides. Lightly brush the pear flesh with olive oil. Place the chicken on the pan, and grill each side for 5 to 7 minutes, or until the chicken is no longer pink (depending on thickness).

Remove the chicken from the pan and let it rest. Place the pears in the pan, flesh side down. Grill for 3 to 4 minutes, or until grill marks are visible. Remove the pears from the pan and let them rest.

In the meantime, to a small bowl, add the coarse ground mustard, Dijon mustard, honey, apple cider vinegar and pepper. Whisk to mix everything together. Set aside.

To assemble the salad, add the spinach, raspberries, red onion, pecans and goat cheese to a large bowl. Slice the chicken and pears and top the salad. Serve with dressing on the side.

*See image on page 54.

SALAD

1 lb (450 g) boneless, skinless chicken breast

Black Pepper, to taste

1 tsp olive oil (avocado or canola would work, too)

Bartlett pear, halved

6 cups (180 g) baby spinach

¾ cup (92 g) raspberries

1 cup (160 g) red onion, sliced

½ cup (65 g) pecan halves

1 oz (28 g) crumbled goat cheese

DRESSING

4 tsp (15 g) coarse ground mustard

1 tbsp (15 ml) Dijon mustard

1 tbsp (15 ml) honey

1 tbsp (15 ml) apple cider vinegar

Black Pepper, to taste

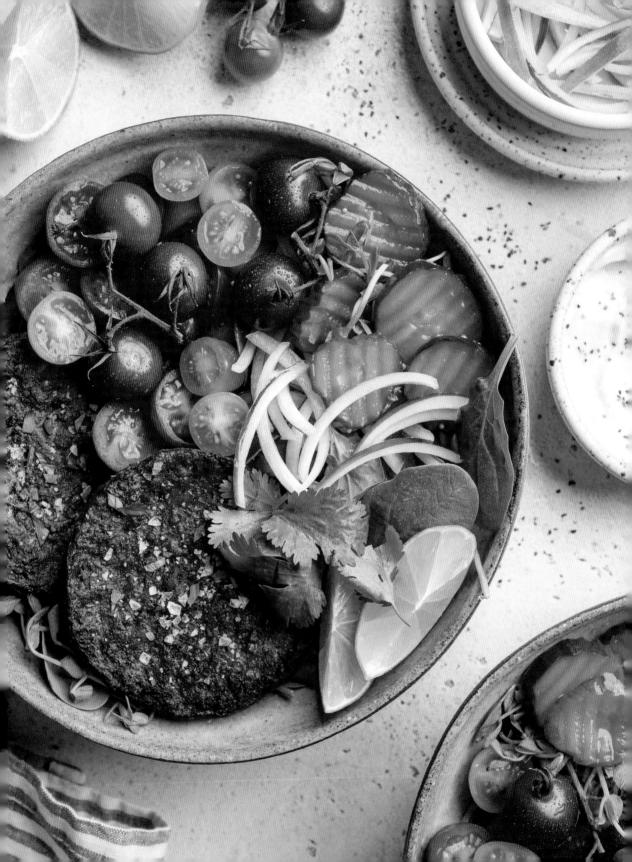

VEGGIE BURGER BOWL

Yield : 1 serving

3⅓ oz (95 g) veggie burger patty of your choice

2 cups (60 g) baby spinach

½ tomato, chopped

¼ cup (40 g) red onion, sliced

½ cup (26 g) pickle of choice, sliced

1 tbsp (15 ml) mayonnaise

Veggie burgers contain a high amount of fiber, which helps to keep you fuller at mealtimes. In addition, higher-fiber intake reduces breast and colon cancer risk!

All you need for this amazing lunch is to cook the veggie burger patty according to package directions. Cut it into slices, then arrange the veggie burger, spinach, tomatoes, red onions and pickles in a bowl and mix in the mayonnaise.

SALMON CHOPPED SALAD

Yield: 1 serving

2 cups (403 g) romaine hearts, chopped

¼ cup (37 g) red bell pepper, chopped

¼ cup (119 g) chopped cucumber

⅛ cup (20 g) chopped red onion

¼ cup (55 g) canned wild salmon, drained and broken into chunks

1 tbsp (3 g) fresh dill, finely chopped

1 tbsp (4 g) fresh parsley, finely chopped

Italian dressing of your choice, to taste

1 slice whole wheat toast

There are many benefits of having a variety of greens in your life. A health benefit of all types of lettuce includes strong bones. Lettuce is a source of vitamin K, which helps strengthen bones. It is hydrating, considering it is 95 percent water. Lettuce is a source of vitamin A and thus supports healthy vision.

Mix the romaine, bell pepper, cucumber, red onion, salmon, dill, parsley and Italian dressing together in a bowl. Serve with a slice of whole wheat toast.

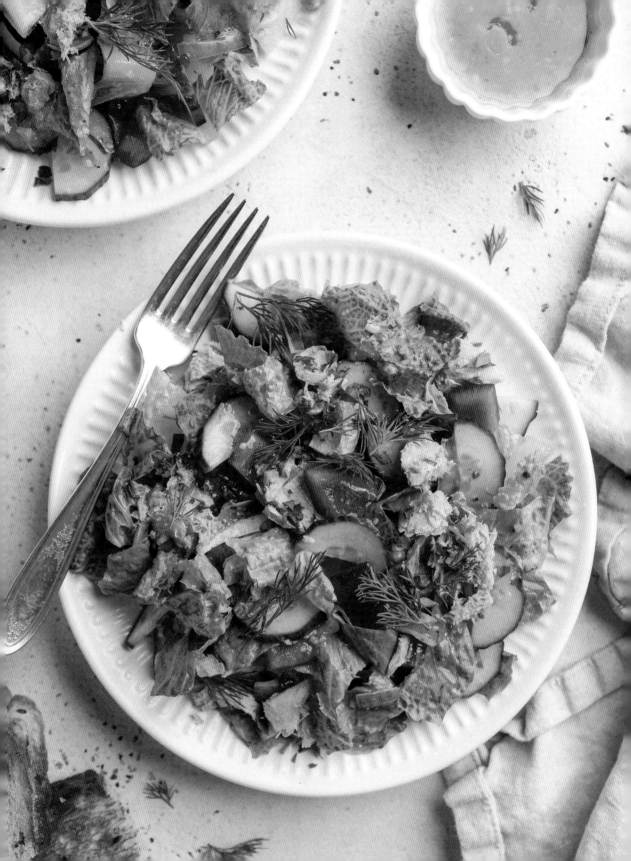

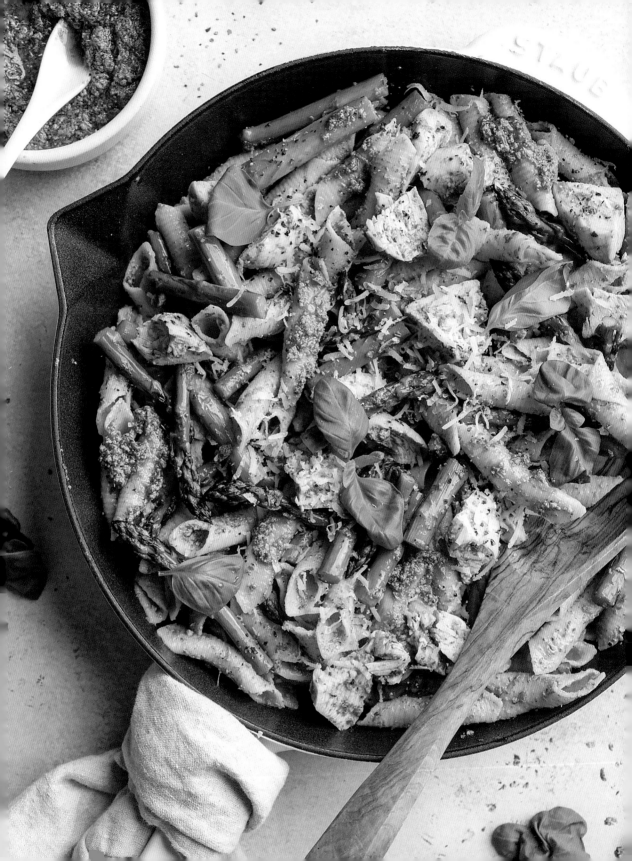

CHICKEN AND ASPARAGUS PESTO PASTA

Yield : 2 servings

8 oz (227 g) chicken breast

2 cups (360 g) raw asparagus, ends trimmed

1 tbsp (15 ml) extra virgin olive oil

9¾ oz (276 g) chickpea rotini pasta, dry

⅓ cup (80 ml) basil pesto

1 tbsp (15 ml) lemon juice

3 tbsp (6 g) Parmigiano-Reggiano, finely grated

Black pepper, to taste

I love a simple and easy lunch that the whole family can enjoy! In this recipe asparagus is a star veggie. Asparagus is a good source of folate, and research shows that foods high in folate help protect against pancreatic, esophageal and bowel cancer. Asparagus is also a source of fiber, and there is evidence that foods containing dietary fiber help protect against bowel cancer. Asparagus is low in calories, like most other vegetables, which can help to support a healthy body weight. Eating at least five servings of vegetables a day helps maintain a healthy weight, which is one of the most important things you can do to reduce your risk of several common cancers. So include asparagus in your diet, along with a variety of vegetables!

Preheat the oven to 400°F (205°C), and line a baking sheet with parchment paper. Add the chicken and asparagus to the baking sheet and drizzle with the oil. Bake for 25 minutes, or until the chicken is cooked through to an internal temperature of 165°F (74°C). Chop the chicken and asparagus into bite-sized pieces.

Meanwhile, cook the pasta according to the package instructions.

To assemble the pasta, mix the chicken, asparagus, pasta, pesto, lemon juice and cheese together. Season with pepper. Divide evenly between bowls and serve.

GREEK EGG AND VEGGIE BOWL

Yield: 1 serving

2 eggs
2 cups (40 g) arugula
¼ tomato, cut into wedges
¼ medium cucumber, diced
¼ cup (40 g) red onion, sliced
¼ medium green bell pepper, sliced
¼ cup (45 g) pitted Kalamata olives
1 tbsp (15 ml) extra virgin olive oil
Salt, to taste
Black pepper, to taste
2 tbsp (19 g) feta cheese, crumbled
½ tsp oregano

Do eggs cause cancer? No, eating eggs does not cause cancer. Studies have looked at the relationship between eggs and different types of cancer, but there is no evidence that eggs affect cancer risk. Eggs can provide a source of protein as part of a healthy, balanced diet! In addition to this delicious egg and veggie bowl, here are some other suggestions for how to combine eggs with plant-based foods to reduce cancer risk:

- Scramble eggs with veggies.
- Serve eggs with whole grain tortillas or whole wheat bread.
- Pair hard-boiled eggs with fruit and whole grain crackers for a hardy snack.
- Pair cottage cheese or other cheese with your scrambled eggs to increase protein intake.

Bring a medium-sized pot of water to a boil and add the eggs. Boil for 7 to 8 minutes, then immediately remove them and place them in ice water.

Meanwhile, prepare the bowl by adding the arugula, tomato, cucumber, onion, bell pepper and olives. Drizzle with the oil. Add salt, pepper and the feta cheese.

Peel the eggs, slice them in half and add them to the bowl. Top with the oregano.

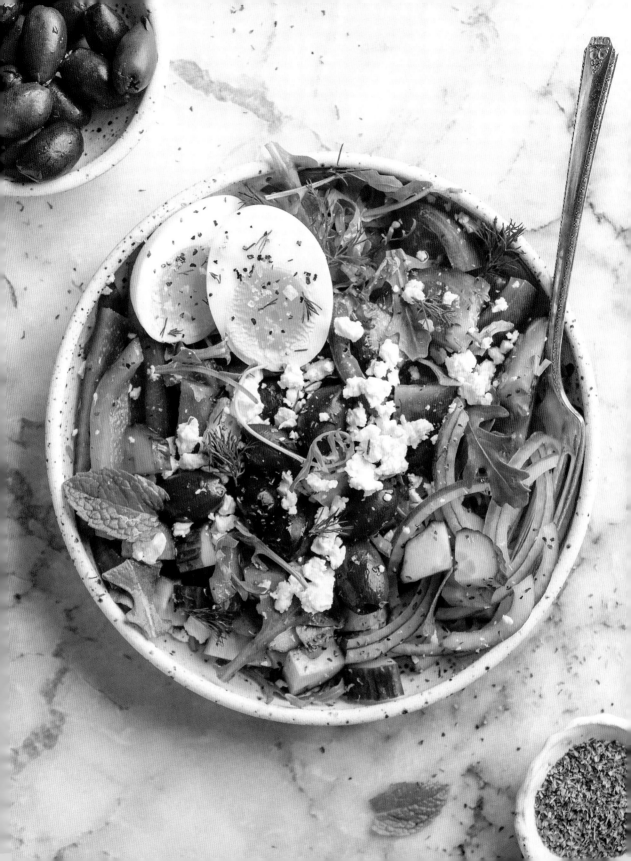

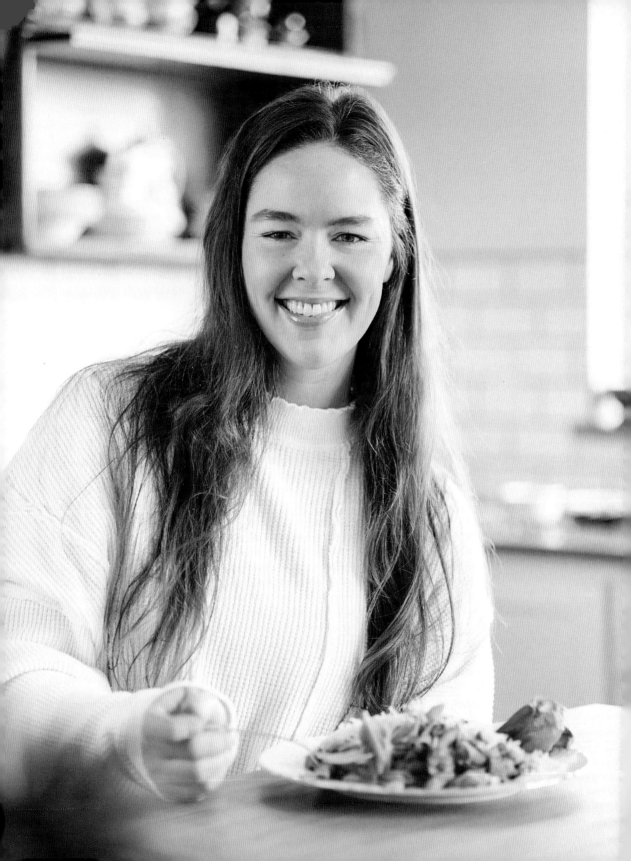

QUICK, NUTRIENT-PACKED
Dinners

Let's simplify dinners while we also reduce cancer risk! Get ready for easy flavor, without the sodium or unhealthy fats. Cancer prevention should be easy, taste good and keep to ingredients that nourish your mind and body. These guidelines are what you can expect the recipes in this chapter to reflect. Oftentimes survivors are told they must shift their diet to "all plants," "no meats" or similar restrictions, but that is not the case. You CAN have meat and reduce cancer risk. That is why you will find a nice assortment of plant-based and meat-based recipes—an enjoyable variety that you can eat with confidence and has ingredients the whole family will love. Remember, you can add in more veggies if you feel up to it. I cannot wait for you to see how simple and flavorful cancer-prevention meals can be!

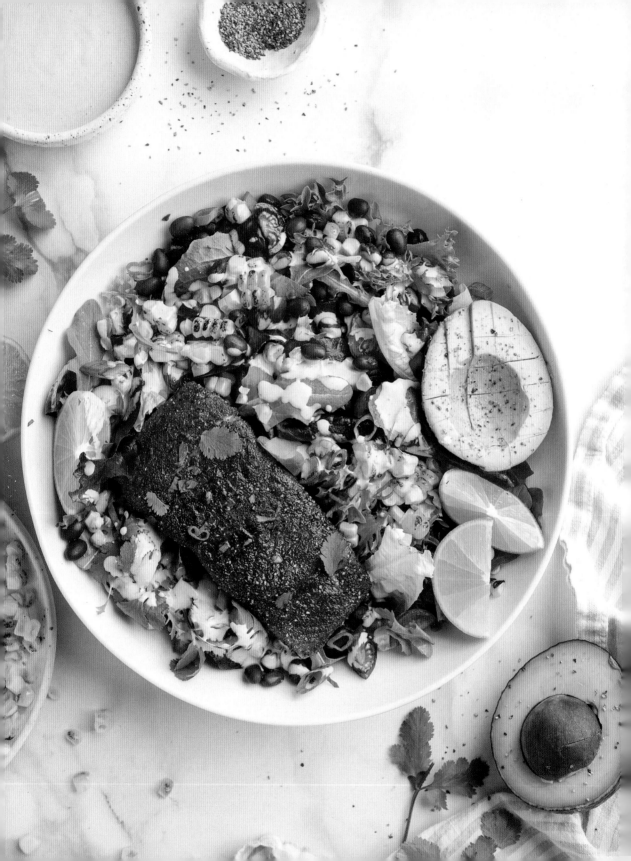

BLACKENED SALMON SALAD WITH CHIPOTLE RANCH DRESSING

Yield : 4 servings

SALMON

1 tsp paprika

1 tsp ground cumin

½ tsp onion powder

½ tsp garlic powder

1 tsp chili powder

¼ tsp black pepper

1 lb (450 g) skinless salmon filets

2 tbsp (30 ml) vegetable or canola oil

SALAD

6 cups (252 g) spring mix lettuce

1 medium avocado, pitted and diced into ½-inch (1.3-cm) cubes

1 medium tomato, diced into ¼-inch (½-cm) cubes

¼ cup (12 g) sliced scallions

1 (15-oz [425-g]) can low-sodium black beans, drained and rinsed

1 (15-oz [425-g]) can low-sodium corn, drained and rinsed

2 tbsp (2 g) minced cilantro

The vitamin B12 in salmon keeps blood and nerve cells humming, but the true beauty of salmon is its wealth of omega-3 fatty acids. Most omega-3s are "essential" fatty acids. Your body can't make them, but they play critical roles in good health. They can reduce the risks of cancer and cardiovascular disease. I recommend that all adults eat at least two portions (a total of 8 ounces [227 g]) of seafood a week, especially fish that are high in omega-3s, like salmon.

To make the salmon, combine all the spices in a small bowl. Then rub the spice mixture evenly all over your salmon filets. In a large nonstick skillet over medium-high heat, heat the vegetable oil for about 3 minutes, until shimmery. Add the salmon to the pan, and sear for 3 to 4 minutes on each side, flipping once until the salmon is cooked through. Remove the salmon from the pan, and set the filets aside to cool while you prepare the salad and dressing.

To make the salad, combine the ingredients in a large bowl. Divide among four serving bowls. Arrange your cooked salmon filets on top, then set aside.

(continued)

BLACKENED SALMON SALAD WITH CHIPOTLE RANCH DRESSING (CONT.)

Make the dressing by combining all ingredients in a blender (or food processor) and blend until completely smooth. Season the dressing with pepper to taste. Drizzle the dressing over the assembled salads and serve immediately.

DRESSING

¼ cup (60 ml) mayonnaise

⅓ cup (80 ml) light sour cream

1 tbsp (15 ml) 2% or skim milk

1 tbsp (15 g) minced chipotle peppers in adobo sauce

1 tbsp (15 g) reserved adobo sauce

¼ tsp garlic powder

¼ tsp onion powder

Black Pepper, to taste

LOADED QUINOA TACOS

Yield : 4 servings (3 tacos per serving)

2 cups (360 g) quinoa

2 cups (473 ml) low-sodium vegetable broth

1 bell pepper

Juice from 1 lime, divided

Ready for another delicious and easy vegetarian dinner idea? Meet a favorite in my household: Loaded Quinoa Tacos! It's a delicious plant-based and vegetarian taco recipe that takes only 30 minutes to make! The quinoa taco "meat" is topped with a quick bell pepper slaw and sour cream. It's magical, vegetarian protein goodness! Let's get started!

In a dry pot over medium heat, add the dry quinoa and toast it, stirring frequently. After a few minutes you'll start to hear a popping sound; continue stirring until the quinoa just starts to brown and smell toasty, 3 to 4 minutes total.

Immediately transfer the quinoa to a fine mesh strainer and rinse it in the sink. Return it to the pot and add the vegetable broth. Bring it to a boil, then reduce the heat to low. Cover the pot, and simmer until the broth is bubbling for 15 to 20 minutes and the broth has been completely absorbed. (Check by pulling back the quinoa with a fork to see if broth remains.) Turn off the heat and let it sit with the lid on to steam for 5 minutes, then fluff the quinoa with a fork.

While the quinoa cooks, make a quick bell pepper slaw: Thinly slice the pepper, then cut the slices in half. Place them in a bowl, and mix with 1 tablespoon (15 ml) of lime juice. Allow the peppers to stand until ready to serve.

(continued)

LOADED QUINOA TACOS (CONT.)

3 tbsp (45 ml) olive oil

1 tbsp (8 g) cumin

1 tbsp (8 g) paprika

1 tsp garlic powder

1 tsp onion powder

1 tsp oregano

2 scallions, sliced

12 corn tortillas

4 cups (168 g) spring mix lettuce

Pickled red onions or jalapeños, to taste (optional)

Light sour cream, to taste

Hot sauce, to taste (optional)

Feta cheese crumbles, to taste

Salsa, to taste (optional)

When the quinoa is done, heat the olive oil in a large nonstick pan over medium heat. Add the cooked quinoa, and stir to combine. Add the cumin, paprika, garlic powder, onion powder and oregano, and stir. Then cook without stirring for about 5 minutes, or until the bottom starts to get crispy. Remove from the heat and stir in 1 tablespoon (15 ml) of lime juice and the scallions. (Add any remaining lime juice to the bell pepper slaw.)

Warm the tortillas by placing a tortilla on an open gas flame on medium for a few seconds per side, flipping with tongs, until slightly blackened and warm. Top the tortillas with the greens, quinoa filling, bell peppers, pickled onions, sour cream (mixed with a little hot sauce if desired), feta crumbles and salsa. Serve immediately.

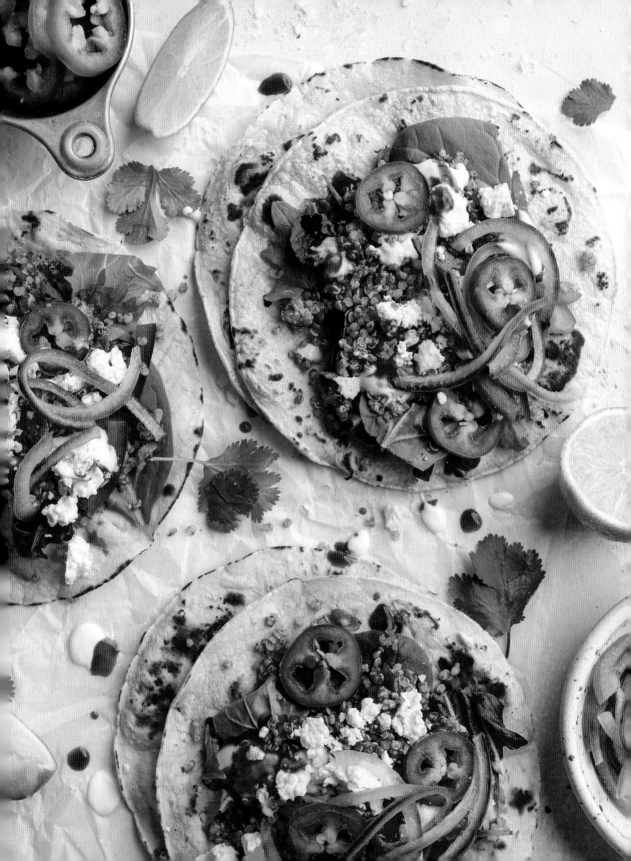

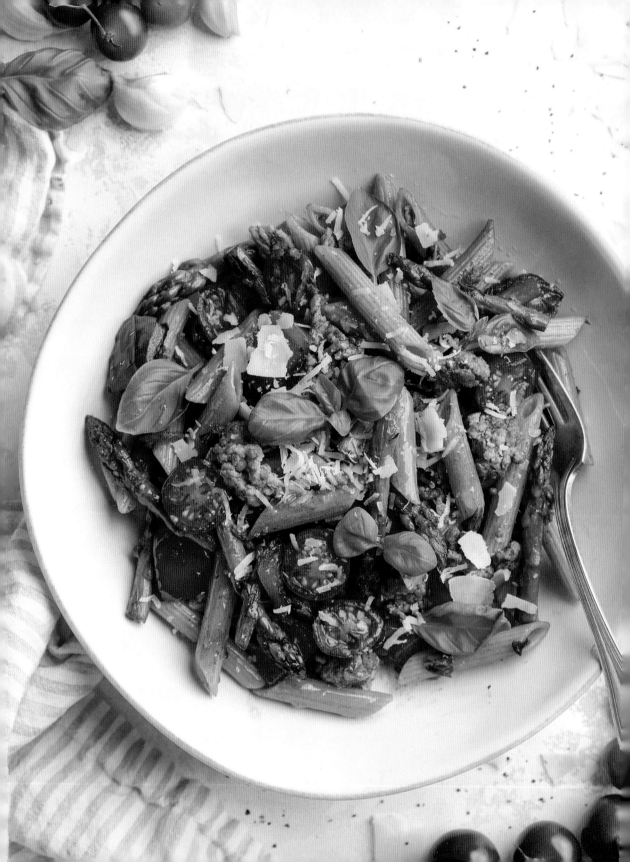

PENNE PASTA WITH VEGGIES AND CRUMBLED TURKEY SAUSAGE

Yield: 4 servings

2 tbsp (30 ml) extra virgin olive oil

1 lb (454 g) lean ground turkey

½ cup (80 g) red onion, grilled and coarsely chopped

½ cup (75 g) red bell pepper, grilled and coarsely chopped

½ cup (90 g) asparagus, grilled and cut into 1-in (2.5-cm) pieces

½ cup (75 g) cherry tomatoes, sliced in half

3 cloves garlic, finely diced

2 tbsp (30 ml) balsamic vinegar

¼ cup (5 g) fresh basil, coarsely chopped, plus more for serving

6 cups (1.2 kg) cooked whole grain penne pasta

Black Pepper, to taste

½ cup (45 g) coarsely grated Parmesan cheese

If you love the pungent flavor and scent of garlic, you are on trend. Cultures have long used garlic both for cooking and medicine. Here in the United States, garlic popularity has soared over the years. That's potentially good news for overall health and a lowered cancer risk. Eating garlic frequently lowers the risk of colorectal cancers. There are many ways in which garlic and its compounds may do this: Lab studies show that garlic compounds help with DNA repair, slowing the growth of cancer cells and decreasing inflammation. Each clove of garlic is full of a variety of phytochemicals, many showing cancer-fighting properties! One of these is flavonoid, which is a compound well studied for its anti-cancer properties.

In a medium saucepan, add the olive oil and cook the ground turkey until lightly brown, about 5 minutes. Then add the onion, pepper, asparagus, cherry tomatoes and garlic. Sauté gently until the mixture is hot and the flavors have married, about 5 minutes. Add the vinegar and the basil.

Add the cooked pasta to the hot mixture. Add pepper to taste.

Place in a large serving dish. Top with the grated cheese and more of the basil.

CHICKPEA PASTA WITH SPINACH

Yield: 3 servings

8 oz (227 g) rotini chickpea pasta

2 tbsp (30 ml) olive oil, divided

1 (15-oz [425-g]) can chickpeas, drained and rinsed

3 cloves garlic, minced

¼ tsp red pepper flakes

½ tsp black pepper

Juice and zest of 1 lemon

1 cup (30 g) torn baby spinach

¼ cup (25 g) grated Pecorino-Romano cheese, plus more for serving

2 tbsp (8 g) chopped parsley

With spinach, lemon, garlic and Pecorino, this super easy chickpea pasta recipe is ready in about 20 minutes. It's vegetarian and gluten-free. To put it simply, chickpeas are the absolute best! Whether at their most basic and dried or at their most convenient and canned, with some straightforward, easy cooking, you can create something pretty great. Chickpeas are high in protein and make an excellent replacement for meat in many vegetarian and vegan dishes. Chickpeas contain a moderate amount of calories and several vitamins and minerals. They're also a good source of fiber!

Cook the pasta in a large pot of boiling salted water until al dente according to the package instructions. Drain and rinse in a fine mesh strainer. Heat 1 tablespoon (15 ml) of olive oil in a large skillet over medium heat and set aside the second tablespoon. Add the chickpeas and sauté, occasionally stirring them. They will turn crispy and golden in 5 to 6 minutes.

Next add the garlic, red pepper flakes and black pepper, cooking for 30 seconds to 1 minute until fragrant. Stir in the pasta, lemon juice, lemon zest and the reserved tablespoon (15 ml) of olive oil. Add the spinach, cheese and parsley. The greens will wilt in a couple minutes. Top with additional cheese before serving.

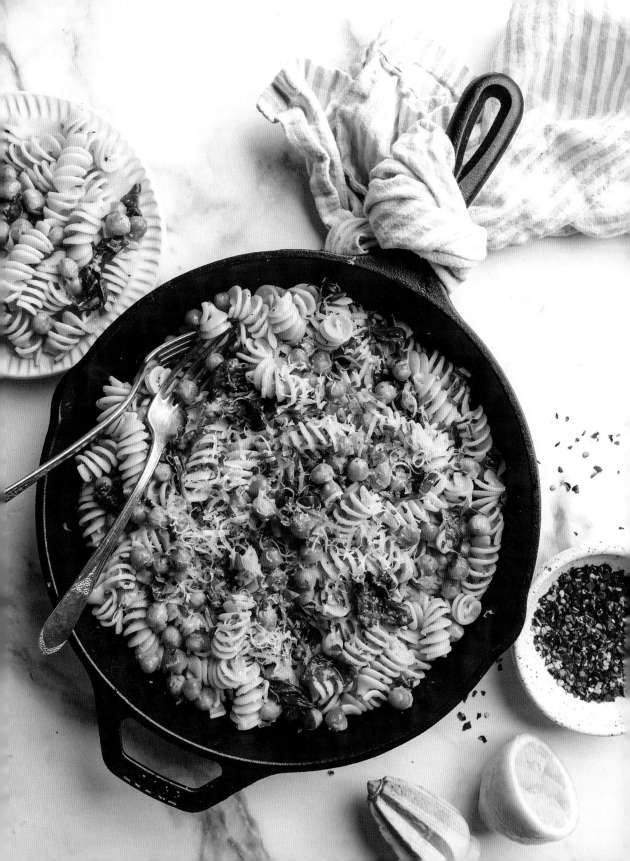

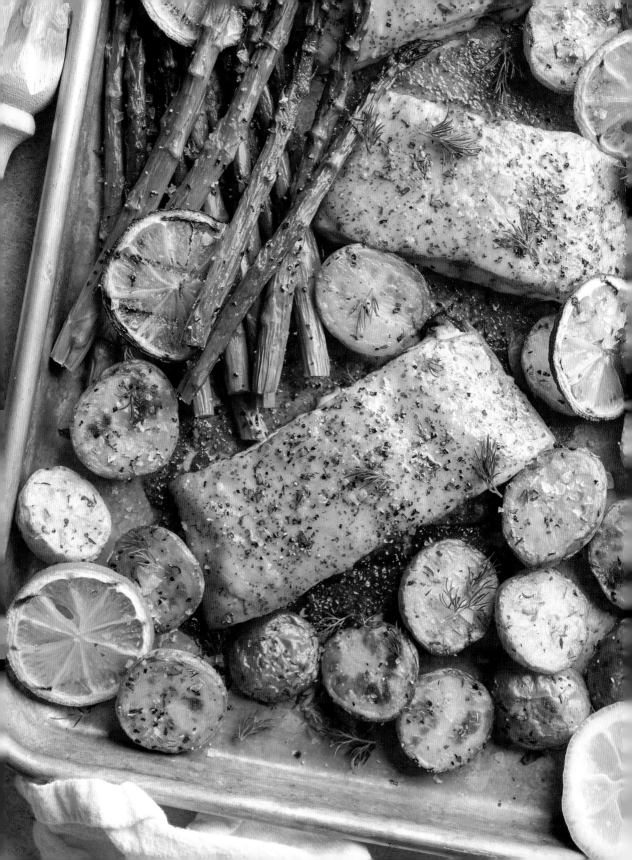

SHEET PAN SALMON AND ASPARAGUS WITH POTATOES

Yield : 4 servings

2 lb (908 g) baby red or gold potatoes, quartered

3 tbsp (45 ml) olive oil, divided

2½ tsp (2 g) Italian herbs, divided

1 tsp garlic powder

Black Pepper, to taste

4 salmon filets

1 lb (454 g) asparagus, ends trimmed

2 tbsp (30 ml) butter, melted

2 tbsp (30 ml) honey

1 tsp Dijon mustard

½ lemon, thinly sliced

Sheet Pan Salmon and Asparagus with Potatoes is a great way to get in a serving of protein and heart-healthy omega-3s. Everyone in your family will love this dish for the flavor, and you'll love it for its ease of cooking and cleanup. I love salmon for many reasons. It's delicious and works so well in all sorts of preparations and marinades. It's one of my family's favorite fish. It's also really healthy for you, and it's easy to purchase from your grocer's fish department, in bulk at the warehouse stores or in the freezer section. For a DIY Italian herb blend, stir together equal parts dried thyme, parsley, oregano and basil.

Preheat the oven to 400°F (205°C). Toss the potatoes with 2 tablespoons (30 ml) of olive oil. Season with 2 teaspoons (2 g) of Italian herbs, the garlic powder and pepper to taste. Arrange them on a large sheet pan, and bake for 10 minutes.

Arrange the salmon filets and asparagus on the sheet pan. Whisk together the melted butter, honey, Dijon mustard and the remaining ½ teaspoon of the Italian herb blend. Brush the mixture onto the salmon filets.

Drizzle the asparagus with the remaining 1 tablespoon (15 ml) of olive oil, then season with pepper to taste and place the lemon slices between the asparagus spears.

Bake for 15 minutes, until the asparagus and potatoes are fork-tender and the salmon is cooked through. Serve immediately.

BEEF TACO RICE BOWL WITH CABBAGE

Yield : 2 servings

½ cup (100 g) brown rice, uncooked
8 oz (225 g) extra-lean ground beef
2 tsp (2 g) taco seasoning
2 tsp (10 ml) avocado oil
3 cups (267 g) purple cabbage, chopped
1 avocado, mashed
2 scallions, chopped
Black pepper, to taste

Protein supports energy levels and treatment recovery! While huge amounts of red meat is not recommended on a cancer-prevention lifestyle, lean ground beef is a good option to include in moderate amounts in your rotation. It's lower in saturated fat and provides a lot of protein for recovery during treatment. This recipe also features purple cabbage, an anthocyanin powerhouse (the same antioxidant found in blueberries).

Cook the rice according to the package directions. Then preheat a frying pan over medium heat. Add the beef, breaking it up as it cooks. Add the taco seasoning, and continue to break up the beef. Cook for 7 to 10 minutes, or until cooked through. In a separate pan, add the oil and sauté the cabbage for 3 to 5 minutes. Divide the rice, beef, cabbage, avocado and scallions evenly between two bowls. Season with pepper.

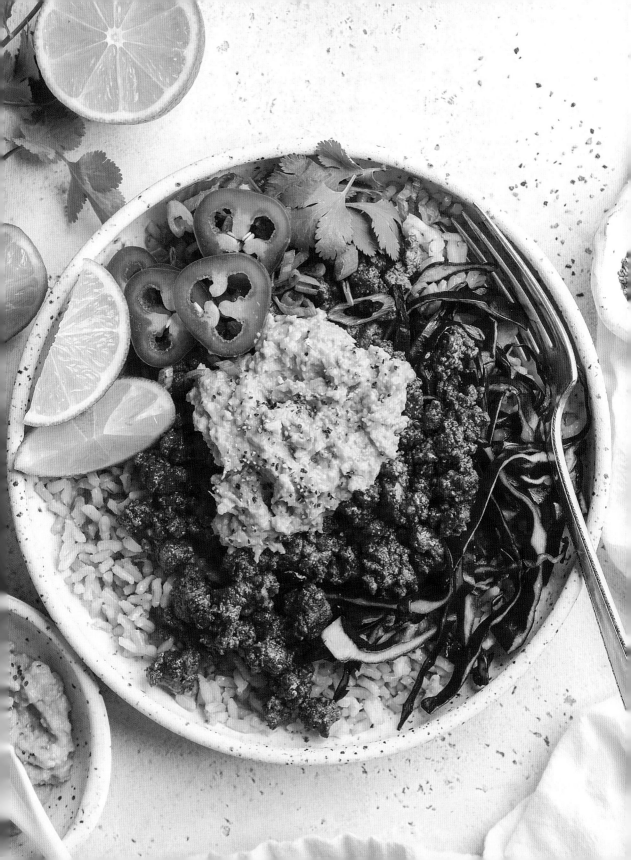

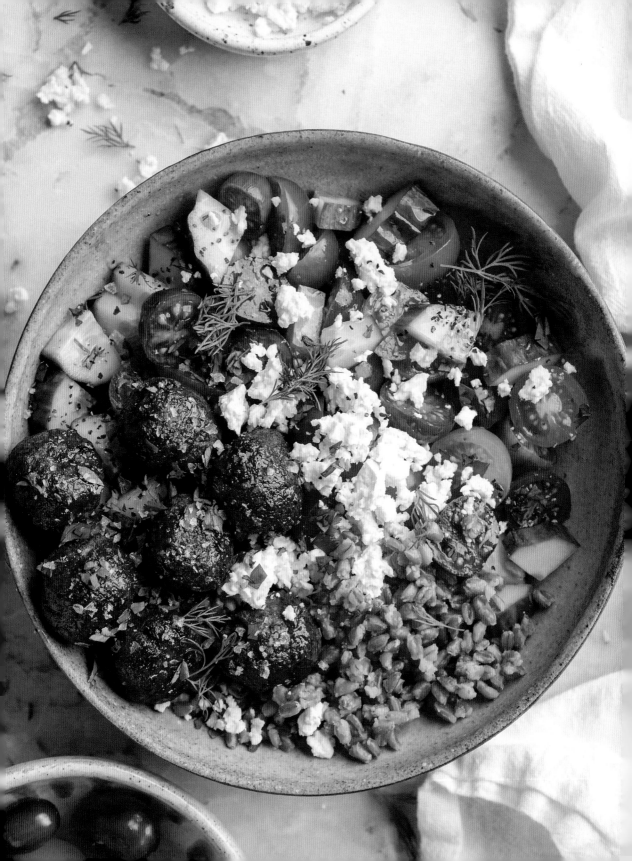

FARRO AND CUCUMBER SALAD WITH MEATBALLS

Yield: 4 servings

1 cup (201 g) farro, uncooked, rinsed
¼ cup (59 ml) extra virgin olive oil, divided
2 tsp (10 ml) white vinegar
Salt
Black pepper
1 lb (450 g) lean ground beef
1½ cups (224 g) cherry tomatoes, halved
¼ medium-sized cucumber, chopped
⅓ cup (50 g) feta cheese, crumbled

Farro is an ancient grain that has been around for many years, and more recently it has grown in popularity. It not only tastes great but is also healthy. It is packed full of fiber, protein, vitamins, minerals and antioxidants, all of which support a cancer-prevention lifestyle. Farro can easily be added to your diet! A few suggestions for serving farro are in salads, soups and warm breakfast bowls.

Cook the farro according to the package directions.

While the farro is cooking, make the dressing by combining 2 tablespoons (30 ml) of the oil, vinegar and a pinch of salt and pepper in a small bowl. Set aside.

In a bowl, combine the ground beef with a big pinch of salt and pepper, then mix to combine. Roll into approximately 2-inch (5-cm) balls and place them onto a plate.

Heat the remaining 2 tablespoons (30 ml) of oil in a cast-iron skillet or frying pan. Add the meatballs and cook them on all sides until they are browned and cooked through, for 12 to 14 minutes. Work in batches if needed.

Divide the farro, tomatoes, cucumber, meatballs, dressing and feta cheese evenly among four bowls.

VEGGIE AND GOAT CHEESE ZUCCHINI BOATS

Yield : 3 servings

3 medium zucchinis

¼ cup (25 g) shallots, thinly sliced

1 cup (91 g) broccoli florets

¼ cup (45 g) green olives, pitted and sliced

¼ cup (14 g) sun-dried tomatoes, sliced

1 cup (180 g) mixed beans, cooked and rinsed

2 tsp (2 g) Italian seasoning

½ cup (115 g) goat cheese, crumbled

This recipe includes olives, which are very high in vitamin E and other powerful anti-oxidants. Studies show that they are good for heart health and can protect against osteoporosis and cancer. One of the poly-phenols in olives is called oleocanthal. This compound appears to share the same phar-macological activity as ibuprofen and acts as a natural anti-inflammatory. Lowering inflammation in the body will reduce cancer and disease risk.

Preheat the oven to 400°F (205°C) and line a baking sheet with parchment paper.

Cut the zucchinis lengthwise down the middle and scoop out the flesh from the center of each zucchini half. Place the zucchini on the baking sheet, cut side up.

In a bowl, combine the shallots, broccoli, olives, sun-dried tomatoes, mixed beans and Italian seasoning. Spoon the filling into each zucchini boat and top each one with goat cheese.

Bake in the oven for 23 to 25 minutes, or until the cheese is golden and the zuc-chini halves have softened. Divide among three plates.

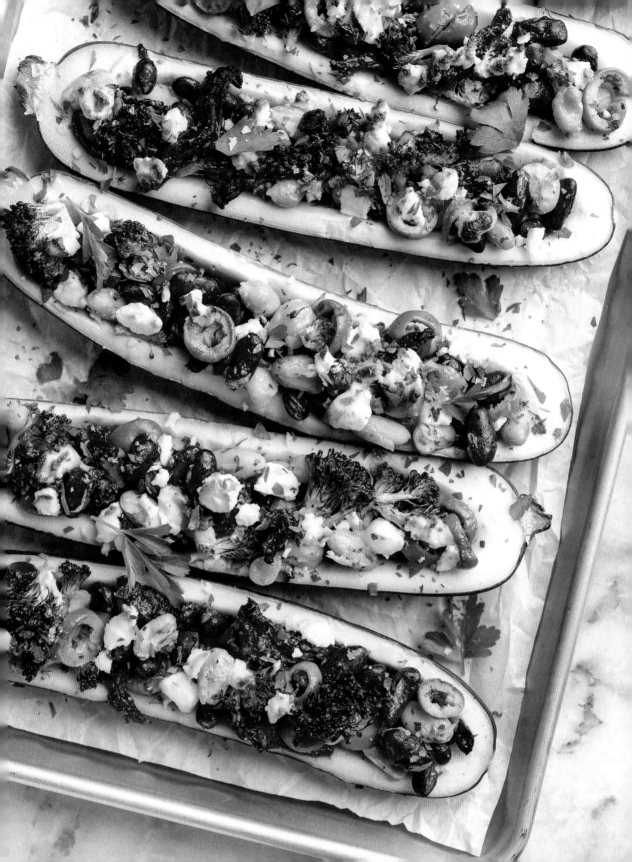

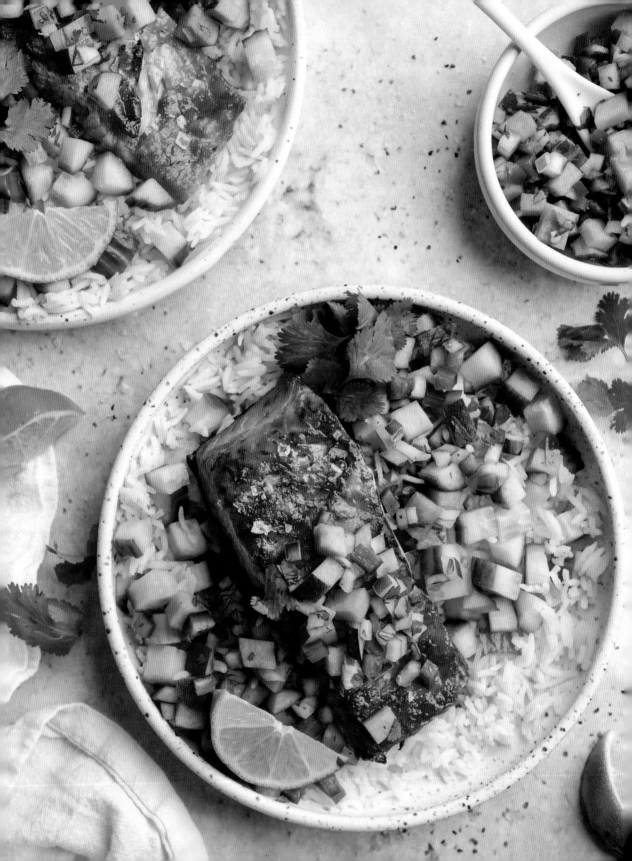

BBQ SALMON BOWL WITH PEACH SALSA

Yield: 2 servings

SALMON BOWL

½ cup (100 g) basmati rice, uncooked

1 tbsp (15 ml) lime juice

12 oz (340 g) salmon filets

½ medium cucumber, finely chopped

SALSA

1 medium peach, finely chopped

¼ cup (40 g) red onion, finely diced

½ jalapeño, finely diced

3 tbsp (3 g) cilantro, finely chopped

1 tbsp (15 ml) lime juice

Peaches are related to plums, apricots, cherries and almonds, all of which reduce cancer risk! They can be eaten on their own or added to a variety of dishes. What's more, peaches are nutritious and may offer an array of health benefits, including improved digestion and healthier skin. Peaches also offer small amounts of magnesium, phosphorus, iron and some B vitamins.

In addition, peaches are packed with antioxidants—beneficial plant compounds that combat oxidative damage and help protect your body against aging and disease. The fresher and riper the fruit, the more antioxidants it contains.

Cook the rice according to the package directions. Preheat your outdoor grill or stovetop grill (or grill pan) to medium heat.

While the rice is cooking, pour the lime juice over the filets and place them on the grill. Cook for 6 minutes on each side.

Meanwhile, make the salsa by combining the peach, red onion, jalapeño, cilantro and lime juice in a bowl. Mix well.

Divide the cucumber, rice, salmon and the peach salsa evenly between two bowls.

TEMPEH, BROWN RICE AND TZATZIKI BOWL

Yield : 2 servings

½ cup (100 g) brown rice, uncooked

2 tsp (10 ml) extra virgin olive oil

6 oz (172 g) tempeh, sliced

1 tbsp (15 ml) balsamic vinaigrette of your choice

¼ cup (37 g) cherry tomatoes, halved

⅛ medium cucumber, quartered and sliced

2 tbsp (16 g) pitted Kalamata olives, chopped

2 tbsp (30 ml) tzatziki sauce of your choice

Tempeh is a versatile ingredient that comes with a variety of health benefits. It's high in protein and prebiotics and contains a wide array of vitamins and minerals. Tempeh is typically made up of fermented soybeans or wheat or both. It can be prepared in a variety of different ways and is high in nutrients, making it a popular vegetarian source of protein: 1 cup (166 g) provides 31 grams of protein and 8 grams of fiber. Wow! Studies show that soy isoflavones also possess antioxidant properties and may reduce oxidative stress as well as the risk of contracting cancer or other diseases. Antioxidants work by neutralizing free radicals. The buildup of harmful free radicals has been associated with many diseases, including diabetes, heart disease and cancer.

Cook the rice according to the package directions.

Heat the oil in a pan over medium-high heat. Add the tempeh and cook until golden, about 4 minutes per side. Remove from the heat. Divide the rice evenly between two bowls. Top with balsamic vinaigrette.

Evenly divide the tempeh, tomatoes, cucumber, olives and tzatziki on top of the rice.

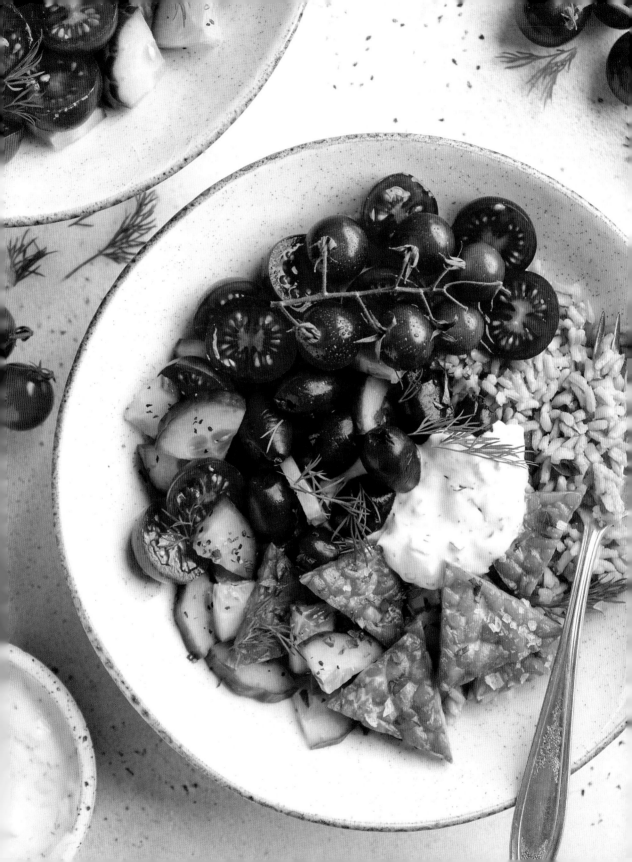

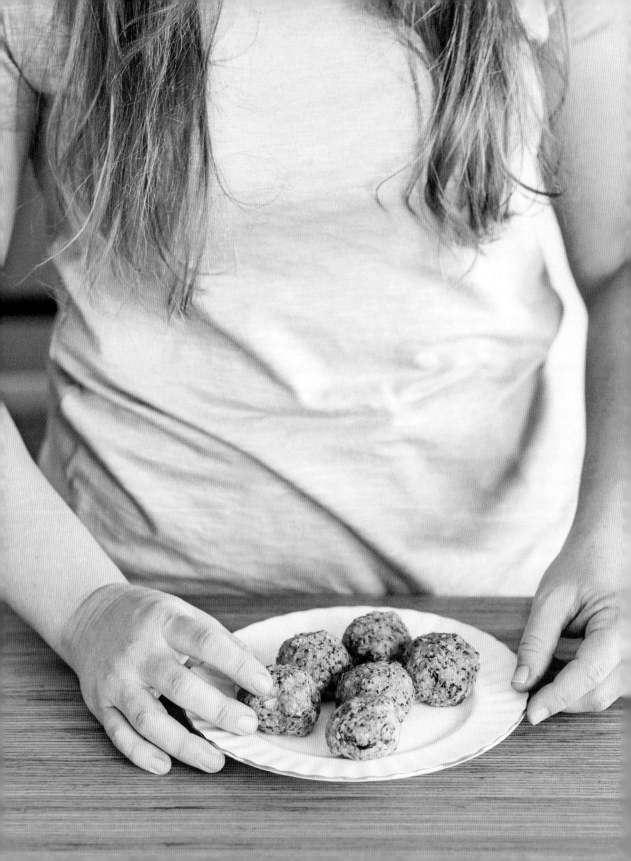

FILLING AND FLAVORFUL
Snacks

Fight off that midday hunger slump with fiber-filled and colorful recipes. So far we have cooked up some inspirational meals, but what about those super fun in-between meal snacks? Did you know that it is actually normal to eat three meals and two to three snacks a day? Yup, you heard me! When we eat throughout the day, we end up feeling more energized, we balance our blood sugars and maintain a healthy body weight, all of which support a healthy and cancer-preventive lifestyle. The amazing snacks in this chapter have a wide variety of flavors, spices and convenience in mind. One key component of these snacks that will really support your cancer-prevention goals is that fiber-rich foods are used in each recipe. Aim to get 30 grams of fiber each day to reduce the risk of colon cancer.

Here are more high-fiber snacking tips and tricks you can also add in to your day:

- Eat your fruit with edible skins on to get all the fiber the plant offers.
- Drink plenty of water! If you consume more than your usual intake of fiber but not enough fluid, you can become constipated. That's because dietary fiber acts like a sponge as it moves through the digestive tract, and thus it needs water to pass through smoothly.
- Eat all the produce you can—all fruits and vegetables are good sources of fiber and antioxidants.
- Carry oat bran or wheat germ with you, and use it as your favorite topping for salads, soups, yogurt and the like.
- Sweeten cereal, oatmeal and baked goods with dried fruit.

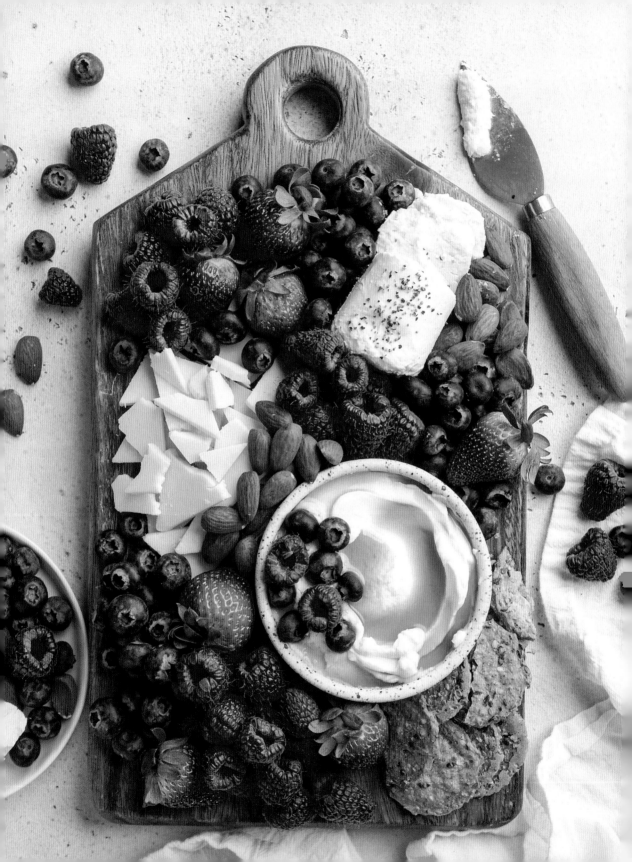

MIXED-BERRY CHEESE BOARD WITH WHIPPED RICOTTA

Yield: 12 servings

¾ cup (185 g) ricotta

1 tbsp (15 ml) honey, plus more for drizzling

The Mixed-Berry Cheese Board with Whipped Ricotta is a berry cheese board filled with strawberries, raspberries, blueberries and the perfect cheeses and nuts to pair with, all of which support a cancer-prevention lifestyle with so much flavor.

Berries contain antioxidants, which help to reduce cancer risk. Studies show these antioxidants protect the body from cell damage that can lead to skin cancer as well as to cancers of the bladder, lung, breast and esophagus. Berries are also a wonderful source of vitamin C, which supports immunity. A serving size of berries is ½ cup (74 g). Other ways to enjoy berries include the following:

- Toss some raspberries in with your morning yogurt or cereal.
- Make a low-fat strawberry smoothie for a quick, healthy snack.
- Bake some delicious oatmeal-blueberry muffins for a meal on the go.

To make the whipped ricotta: Add the ricotta and honey to a food processor and process for 1 to 2 minutes, until totally smooth and creamy, stopping to scrape down the sides of the food processor as needed. Transfer it to a bowl and top with an extra drizzle of honey, as desired.

(continued)

MIXED-BERRY CHEESE BOARD WITH WHIPPED RICOTTA (CONT.)

6 oz (173 g) goat cheese

6 oz (173 g) sharp white Cheddar, sliced

½ cup (72 g) whole strawberries

½ cup (74 g) blueberries

½ cup (62 g) raspberries

Almonds, or nuts of choice, as desired

Whole grain crackers of choice, as desired

Let your creative preparation skills come out with the assembling of the berry cheese board: Grab your favorite cheese board, large dish or platter. I like to start with the cheeses: Slice them and place them around the board, then slice and quarter the strawberries, then add the blueberries, raspberries and almonds, then add the crackers, which should be placed to fill up the board. I find it's easiest to start with the largest components, then fill in the extra spaces throughout the board with the smaller components.

SPICED ZUCCHINI, CARROT AND BANANA BREAD (OR MUFFINS!)

Yield: 12 servings

¾ cup (94 g) all-purpose flour

¾ cup (90 g) whole wheat flour (can also sub another ¾ cup [94 g] all-purpose flour)

1 tsp baking powder

½ tsp baking soda

2 tsp (5 g) cinnamon

½ tsp nutmeg

2 very ripe bananas, mashed

1 large egg

¾ cup (165 g) brown sugar

½ cup (120 ml) vegetable oil

1 tsp vanilla

Enjoy this Spiced Zucchini, Carrot and Banana Bread (or Muffins!) all week long for breakfast, with scrambled eggs, fresh fruit and a smear of your favorite nut butter! One special cancer-prevention ingredient in this amazing recipe is carrots! Carrots, with their rich supply of carotenoids, show the potential to lower the risk of cancer in a variety of well-studied ways. Beta-carotene is the carotenoid that has received the most attention when it comes to reducing the risk of cancer. You can chop carrots or grate them to make a great addition to a variety of dishes. Toss them into vegetable and pasta salads, as well as stews, stir-fries, spaghetti sauce and soup.

Preheat the oven to 350°F (180°C) and prepare a loaf pan or three mini loaf pans with butter or cooking spray. You can also make this recipe into muffins, in which case you would prepare a twelve-tin muffin pan with cooking spray or liners.

In a large bowl, whisk together the flours, baking powder, baking soda, cinnamon and nutmeg. Set aside.

In another bowl, beat together the bananas, egg, sugar, oil and vanilla. You can use a stand mixer, a hand mixer or your own two hands! If you're hand mixing, I suggest using a fork, which seems to work better than a spoon. Mix the wet ingredients with the dry ones until just combined.

(continued)

SPICED ZUCCHINI, CARROT AND BANANA BREAD (OR MUFFINS!) (CONT.)

1 cup (150 g) shredded zucchini, tightly packed
½ cup (55 g) shredded carrot
½ cup (59 g) chopped walnuts

Add the zucchini, carrots and walnuts and stir until incorporated into the batter. It should become easier to mix at this point. Bake for 50 to 60 minutes in the loaf pan (30 to 40 minutes in the mini loaf pan or 18 to 22 minutes in the muffin tin), or until a wooden toothpick comes out clean. Start checking the bread early. Baking times will vary depending on your oven. Let it cool in the pan for 10 to 15 minutes, and then invert and place it on a wire rack to cool completely.

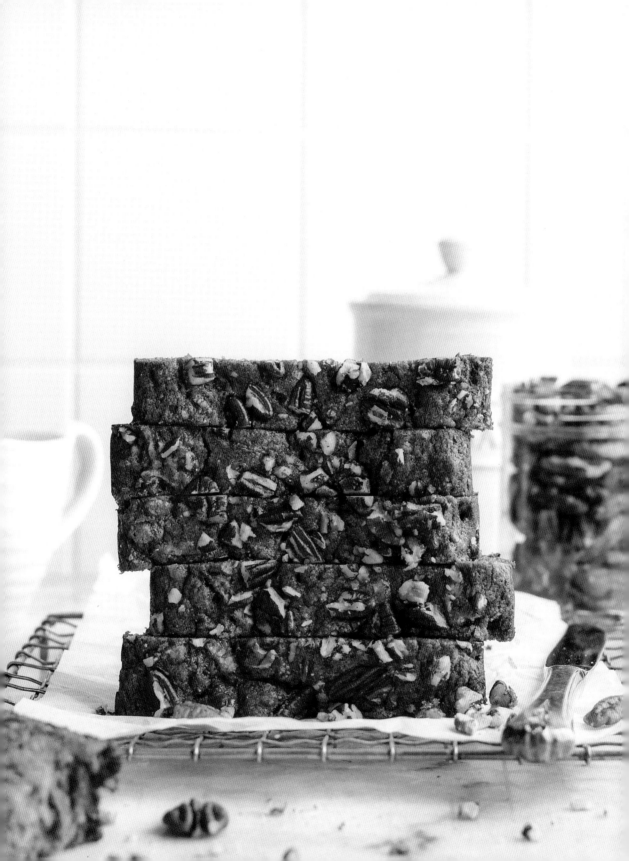

PEANUT BUTTER TOAST WITH BANANA AND CHIA SEEDS

Yield: 2 servings

2 slices of whole wheat bread of choice
Peanut butter, crunchy or creamy, to taste
Honey, for drizzling
½ tbsp (5 g) chia seeds
1 banana

The secret to delectable toast is all in the topping combination. Today I want to share with you how to assemble what I would easily consider to be the ultimate toast topping combination. For this recipe, you'll need a few ingredients that you probably already have in your pantry: your favorite whole wheat bread, bananas, honey and chia seeds. That's it! Let's talk about the powerful benefits of chia seeds. The anti-oxidants, minerals, fiber and omega-3 fatty acids in chia seeds support a cancer-prevention lifestyle and strong bones.

Start by toasting the bread. Then top each slice of toast with the desired amount of peanut butter.

In zigzag motions, drizzle the desired amount of honey.

Next, sprinkle with the chia seeds. Then cut a banana into 18 slices and place them on top of your toast in three rows of three pieces each.

QUICK ENERGY BITES

Yield : 12 bites

⅔ cup (172 g) smooth peanut butter

½ cup (84 g) semi-sweet chocolate chips

¼ cup (35 g) pumpkin seeds, finely chopped

1 cup (90 g) rolled oats

3 heaping tbsp (33 g) raisins, finely chopped

½ cup (60 g) ground seed blend (I use a hemp-chia-flax blend, but if you don't have all three, then use any one of them.)

2 tbsp (30 ml) honey

1 tsp vanilla extract

Here's a little bit about the goodness found in seed energy bites. In this recipe, the flax- and hempseed rank high for omega-3—an essential fat that is excellent for heart and brain function. Hempseed also has the ideal balance of omega-6 to omega-3, which is considered to be an optimal combination for our body. The seeds in this recipe ensure that you receive a good dose of all the essential amino acids. Using a balance of different seeds in your diet, like this, will also ensure a great supply of protein and fiber! These energy bites are jam packed with other nutrients. We're talking phosphorus, magnesium, selenium, manganese, zinc, iron, copper, B vitamins, vitamin K and antioxidant-rich vitamin E (and more). All are essential for supporting healthy organs and cells on multiple levels. What other awesome component of seeds reduce cancer risk? The fiber! Like most plant-based foods, seeds are naturally full of fiber. Fiber is good for blood sugar control, helping to slow the breakdown of carbohydrates and the absorption of sugar. It is also excellent for promoting healthy bowel movements, heart health and weight-loss management.

Combine all the ingredients in a medium bowl. Stir thoroughly. Place in the refrigerator for 15 to 30 minutes so the bites will be easier to roll. Roll into 12 bites and store in the fridge for up to a week.

* See image on page 102.

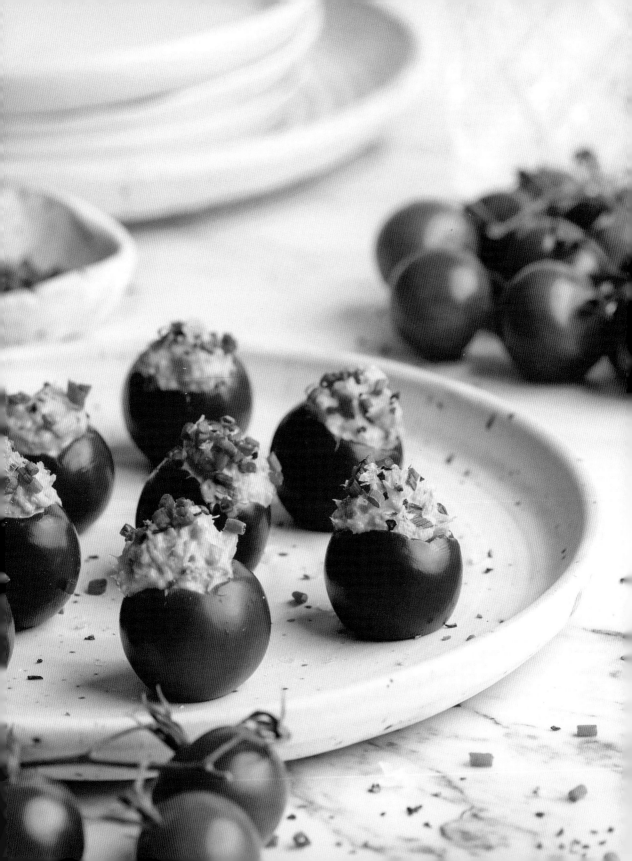

SALMON-STUFFED CHERRY TOMATOES

Yield : 6 servings

2 cups (298 g) whole cherry tomatoes

3¾ oz (105 g) canned wild salmon

1 tbsp (15 ml) mayonnaise

1 tbsp (3 g) chives, chopped

Black pepper, to taste

Tomatoes and salmon are superstars that can reduce cancer risk! Tomatoes are a rare source of lycopene, which is a red-colored carotenoid. Tomatoes can help decrease the risk of bladder, lung and estrogen-receptive cancers. Salmon contains plenty of omega-3 (which improves brain function) and protein (which helps with tissue repair and infection healing), and it's also low in saturated fat.

Cut the tops off of the cherry tomatoes and scoop out the insides using a small spoon. Discard or save for another dish.

Add the salmon, mayonnaise, chives and pepper to a bowl and mix until well combined. Stuff each tomato with the salmon mixture until it is all used up.

POWER SNACK PLATE

Yield : 1 serving

2 eggs, for hard-boiling
1 cup (148 g) blueberries
1 cup (144 g) strawberries, halved
1 oz (18 g) almonds
1 oz (28 g) mozzarella cheese

Almonds contain lots of healthy fats, fiber, protein, magnesium and vitamin E. The health benefits of almonds include lower blood sugar levels, reduced blood pressure and lower cholesterol levels. They can also reduce hunger and promote weight loss.

Place the eggs in a saucepan and cover with water. Bring to a boil over high heat, then turn off the heat but keep the saucepan on the hot burner. Cover and let sit for 10 to 12 minutes.

Transfer the eggs to a bowl of cold water. When the eggs have cooled enough to handle, peel and slice them, and serve with blueberries, strawberries, almonds and cheese on a plate.

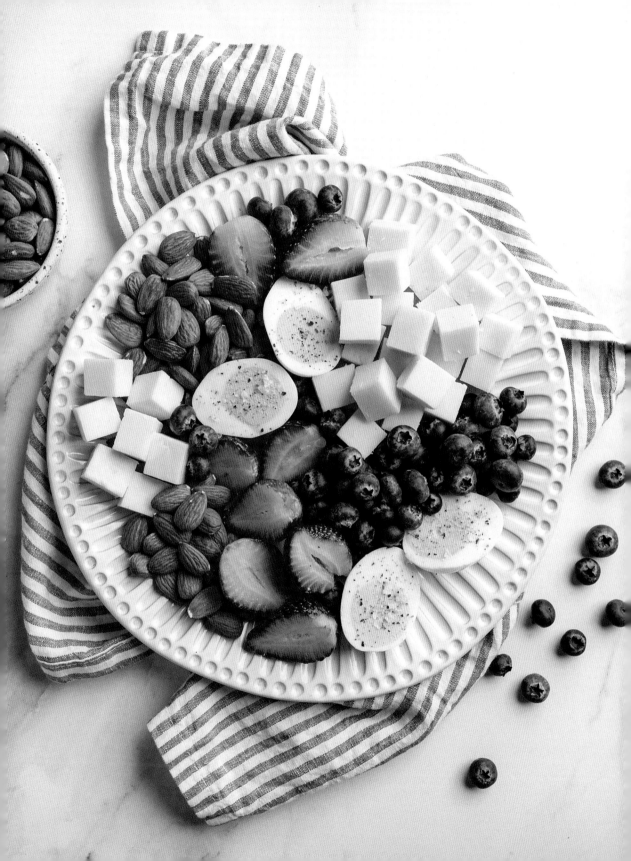

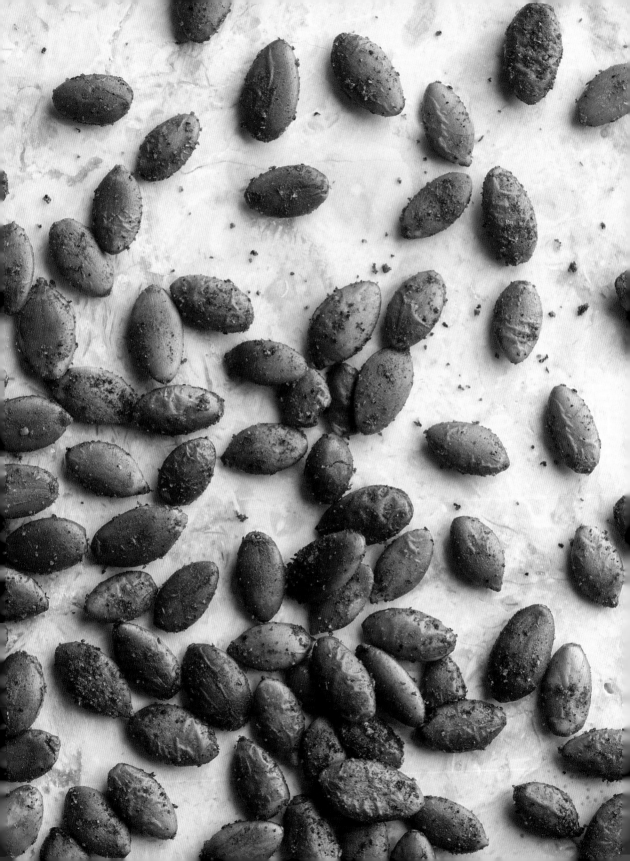

SMOKED BBQ-SPICED PUMPKIN SEEDS

Yield: 12 servings

1½ cups (207 g) raw pumpkin seeds, unshelled

1¼ tsp (4 g) onion powder

¼ tsp ground mustard

1¼ tsp (4 g) garlic powder

½ tsp smoked paprika

¼ tsp cayenne pepper

¼ tsp light brown sugar

1 tsp olive oil

An ounce of Smoked BBQ-Spiced Pumpkin Seeds contains about 151 calories. Pumpkin seeds are a great source of dietary fiber—shelled seeds provide 1.1 grams of fiber in a single 1-ounce (28-gram) serving! Higher-fiber diets help reduce the risk of colon cancer and help to regulate weight. Pumpkin seeds contain antioxidants, including carotenoids and vitamin E. Antioxidants reduce inflammation and protect your cells from harmful free radicals, which is why consuming foods rich in antioxidants can help protect against many diseases and reduce the risk of cancer. Diets rich in pumpkin seeds have been associated with a reduced risk of stomach, breast, lung, prostate and colon cancers. A large observational study found that eating them was associated with a reduced risk of breast cancer in postmenopausal women.

Preheat the oven to 300°F (150°C). Spread the seeds on a baking sheet lined with parchment and roast for about 10 minutes, or until the seeds are dry, tossing halfway through.

In a small bowl, combine the onion powder, ground mustard, garlic powder, smoked paprika, cayenne and sugar.

Place the seeds in a medium bowl and add the olive oil. Add the spice mixture and toss evenly to coat. Spread the seeds evenly on the baking sheet and roast for 20 to 30 minutes, or until brown and crunchy, tossing halfway through.

Remove the pan from the oven and allow the seeds to cool completely before removing to an airtight bag or jar for storage.

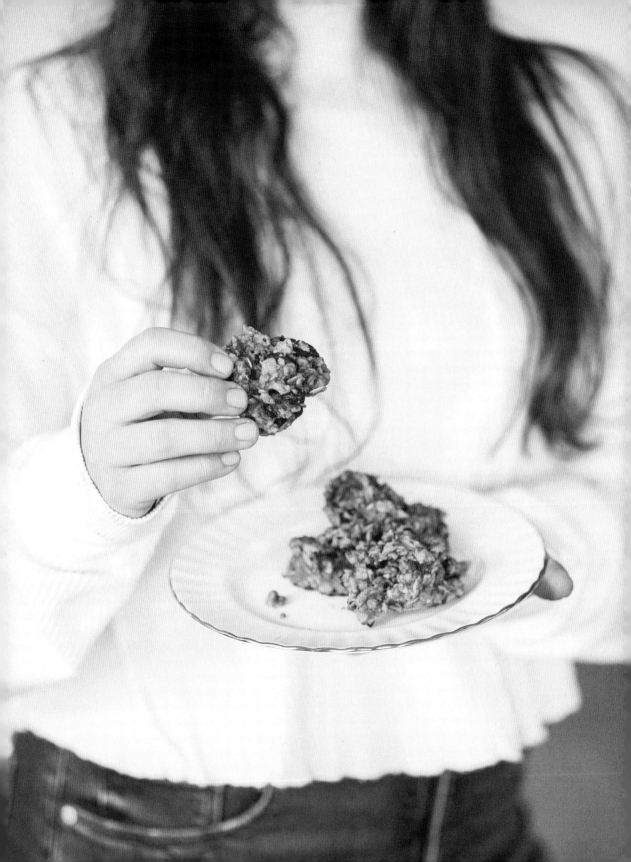

Best-Ever
CANCER-PREVENTION DESSERTS

I love a healthy dessert recipe—it's one of my favorite things to share! I also love being a cancer dietitian who shows you how to dispel your fear of foods, especially when it comes to sugar.

White sugar, brown sugar, cane sugar and the like get a terrible reputation in the wellness world. The same group of people who will claim that sugar is "poison" (it's not!) will nevertheless tell you that you should use maple syrup, coconut sugar, agave or honey because they have more nutrients. Although maple syrup or honey may have "more nutrients," you would have to consume so much of them to obtain the minerals in any substantial quantity that it would negate any health benefits.

(continued)

So what's the deal? The truth is that all sugar, no matter its source, breaks down into the same thing: glucose! There is no need to substitute agave or maple syrup for white sugar unless you prefer the taste! Our bodies do not know if sugar came from a banana, honey or table sugar. How about the phrase "sugar feeds cancer"? As I mentioned earlier, this is a *myth*. Sugar—aka glucose—feeds every single cell in the body. In fact, glucose is the body's preferred source of energy; the brain and red blood cells rely exclusively on glucose! While it is true that cancer cells utilize glucose, having sugar does not make cancer grow quicker.

Even if you were to cut out all sugar (no fun!), the cancer cells would adapt to the new environment and obtain nutrients in other ways, such as by breaking down and converting the protein in your muscle to get the fuel it wants! *Cancer cannot be starved.*

The purpose of this chapter is to get you back to being excited to eat your birthday cake, go on an ice cream outing or enjoy eating your favorite candy bar! I know after cancer you want to make all the right decisions to reduce risk, but you also want to build a life without restriction or bland taste: That is exactly why I have created this dessert chapter for you!

From chocolate treats to fruity desserts, I've got something you'll love! These healthier, sweet treats make for satisfying snacks or post-dinner desserts. Here's to sweet enjoyment!

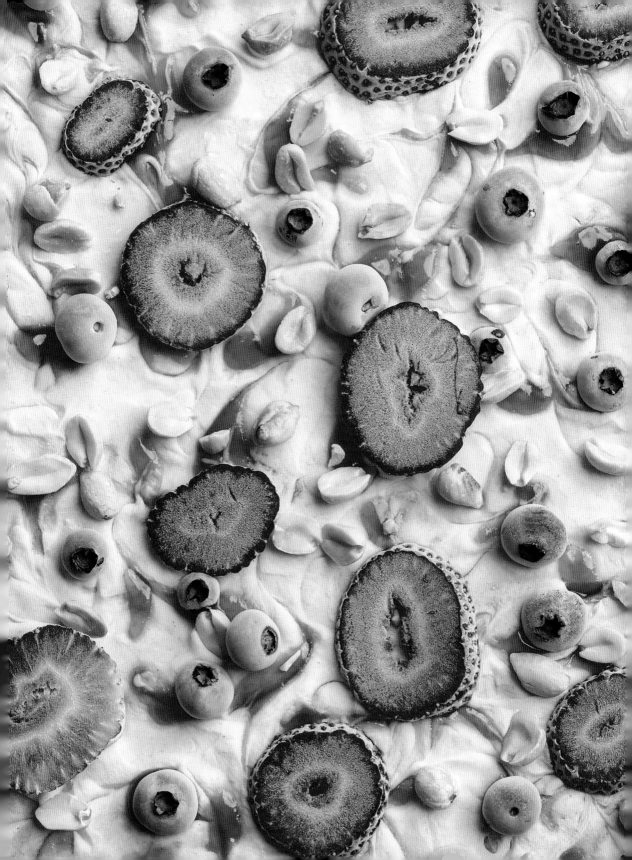

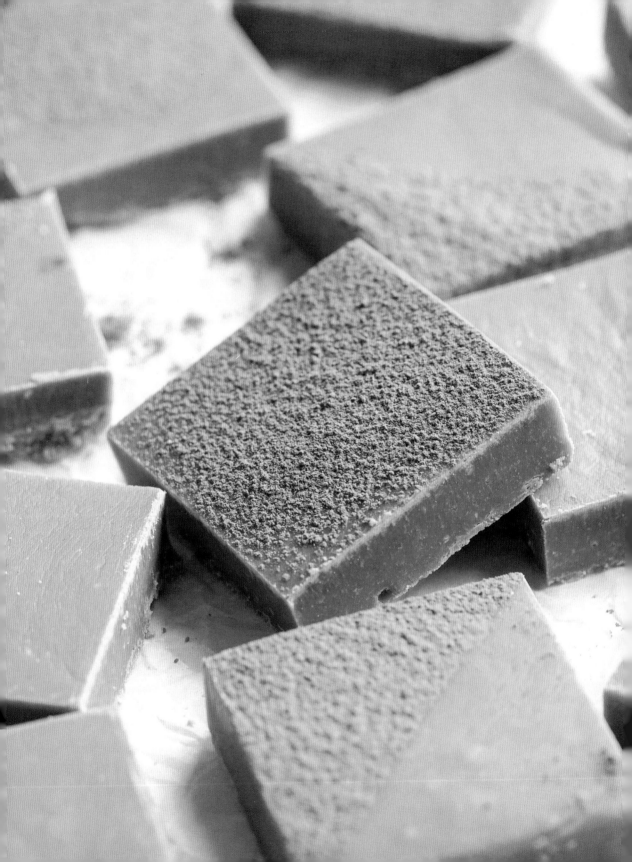

MATCHA FUDGE

Yield : 10 servings

2 tbsp (12 g) matcha powder, plus extra for sprinkling

¾ cup (175 ml) condensed milk

14 oz (397 g) white chocolate chips

1 tsp vanilla extract

Salt, to taste

This matcha fudge is super easy to make and is the perfect quick and flavorful dessert. Matcha is rich in catechins, a class of plant compounds in tea that acts as natural antioxidants. Antioxidants help stabilize harmful free radicals, which are compounds that can damage cells and cause chronic disease or cancer. When you add matcha powder to hot water to make tea, the tea contains all the nutrients from the entire leaf. It will tend to have more catechins and antioxidants than simply steeping green tea leaves in water.

Prepare an 8 x 8-inch (20 x 20–cm) baking pan by covering it with parchment paper. Heat the matcha powder and condensed milk in a saucepan on medium-low until both are well incorporated. Make sure to sift the matcha into the pan. Then, add the white chocolate chips, and mix until they melt. Finally, add the vanilla extract and salt. Mix until incorporated.

Pour the fudge into the prepared baking pan, and use a spatula to spread it into an even layer. Cool at room temperature until fully cool (this will take 15 to 20 minutes). Cover and chill for at least 3 hours in the fridge. If you desire, sift extra matcha powder over the top before serving. Cut into 10 pieces and either serve or store in an airtight container in the fridge for 3 or 4 weeks or at room temperature for up to 2 weeks.

RASPBERRY-VANILLA PROTEIN MUG CAKE

Yield: 1 serving

3 tbsp (24 g) organic buckwheat flour

1 scoop vanilla protein powder of your choice (the average scoop size is 29 g but differs from brand to brand)

½ tsp baking powder

Dash of salt

1 tbsp (15 ml) maple syrup

½ tsp vanilla extract

1 tbsp (16 g) smooth nut butter of your choice

3 tbsp (45 ml) milk of your choice

¼ cup (31 g) fresh or frozen raspberries

Filled with healthy and super-filling ingredients, the Raspberry-Vanilla Protein Mug Cake is the perfect quick, single-serving solution for your sudden sweet cravings. Gluten- and grain-free, organic buckwheat flour has more protein, dietary fiber and B vitamins than an equal weight of oat or whole wheat flour, and it is an excellent source of potassium and essential amino acids.

Add the flour, protein powder, baking powder and salt into a small bowl and mix well. Add the maple syrup, vanilla, nut butter and milk and mix until smooth. Gently fold in the raspberries. Transfer it into a mug and microwave for 2 minutes, or until cooked through, then serve immediately.

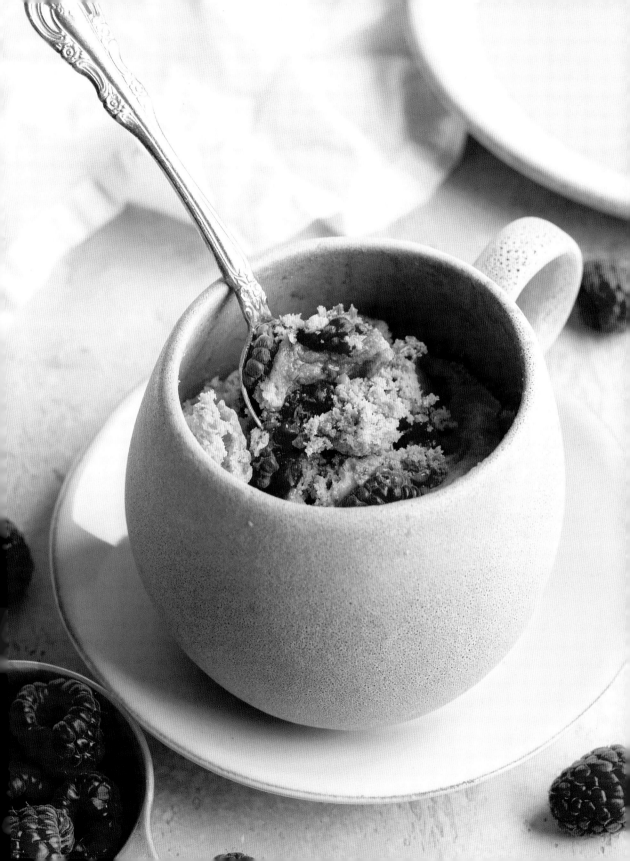

EASY FOUR-INGREDIENT BANANA OATMEAL COOKIES

Yield: 15 cookies

2 bananas, ripe and spotty
1½ cups (135 g) rolled oats
½ cup (129 g) smooth nut or seed butter
⅔ cup (105 g) dark chocolate chips

These Four-Ingredient Banana Oatmeal Cookies are so easy to make in just one bowl. The flavors of banana, oatmeal, peanut butter and chocolate combine to make for a yummy, healthy snack or simple dessert. They are perfect for the whole family! Store leftover cookies in an airtight container at room temperature for 3 to 5 days. To freeze the cookies, place them in an airtight container in the freezer for up to 3 months.

Preheat the oven to 350°F (180°C). Line a large baking sheet with parchment paper, then set aside.

In a large mixing bowl, mash the bananas with a fork until they are soft and creamy. Add the oats and nut butter to the bowl. Stir until a thick dough forms. Fold in the chocolate chips with a rubber spatula or large spoon until they're evenly incorporated throughout the dough.

Use a small cookie scoop to drop even-sized mounds of dough onto the prepared baking sheet. Use your hands or the back of a spatula to flatten the cookies. They do not spread while baking, so make sure they are the right size and shape before you put them in the oven.

Bake the cookies for 10 to 13 minutes, or until the edges are slightly golden brown. Do not overbake them, as they will continue to cook as they cool.

Remove the cookies from the oven, and allow them to cool on the baking sheet for 10 minutes before transferring them to a cooling rack.

* See image on page 118.

BERRY FRUIT KEBABS WITH STRAWBERRY CREAM CHEESE YOGURT DIP

Yield : 4 servings

KEBABS

1½ cups (355 g) cantaloupe chunks

1 cup (144 g) fresh blackberries

1 cup (144 g) fresh strawberries, halved if large

½ fresh pineapple, cored and cut into bite-sized chunks

3 kiwis, peeled and cut into bite-sized pieces

DIP

4 oz (112 g) package of cream cheese, room temperature

¾ cup (112 g) fresh strawberries, stemmed

1 cup (237 ml) vanilla yogurt

3 tbsp (45 ml) honey

I love cooking with my kiddos, and these kebabs are a great way to get them involved in the kitchen. Everyone can choose their own combination of fruit to thread onto the kebabs, and the dip is a great make-ahead recipe that will keep fresh in the refrigerator for several days.

For the fruit kebabs: Thread the cantaloupe, blackberries, strawberries, pineapples and kiwis onto eight 12-inch (30-cm) metal or wooden skewers. Chill until ready to serve.

To make the dip: Put the cream cheese, strawberries, yogurt and honey in a food processor, and pulse until the strawberries are minced and the mixture is smooth. Serve the yogurt dip with the kebabs.

MATCHA-CRANBERRY WHITE CHOCOLATE BARK

Yield: 8 servings

12 oz (340 g) white chocolate baking bars (3 at 4 oz [113 g] each), divided

1 tsp matcha powder

¼ cup (30 g) dried cranberries

2 tbsp (14 g) sliced almonds (optional)

1 tbsp (10 g) chocolate chips (optional)

1 tbsp (11 g) crystallized ginger, chopped (optional)

Make this pretty Matcha-Cranberry White Chocolate Bark to give as gifts, put on your holiday cookie exchange plate or just enjoy it yourself!

Line a small baking sheet with parchment paper and set aside. Place 8 ounces (85 g) of chocolate (2 baking bars, chopped) in a medium glass bowl. Place the remaining chocolate (1 baking bar) in a small glass bowl. Microwave the bowls for 30 seconds on high. Stir the chocolate with a spoon, then return it to the microwave for another 20 to 30 seconds and stir again until it's completely smooth. Repeat in 15-second increments until the chocolate is melted. Alternatively, this can be done in a double boiler or using a glass bowl over a boiling pot of water.

In the small bowl of white chocolate, stir in the matcha until it's evenly dispersed and the matcha chocolate is smooth.

Pour the medium bowl of white chocolate on the lined baking sheet. Using a spatula or large spoon, spread the mixture into a rectangle shape, approximately 8 x 10 inches (20 x 25 cm). Transfer small spoonfuls of the matcha chocolate onto the white chocolate rectangle, then using a toothpick, swirl the white chocolate and matcha chocolate together.

Sprinkle the dried cranberries over the rectangle, and the optional toppings, if using. Gently press the toppings into the chocolate so they set in. Place the chocolate on a baking sheet in the refrigerator for 20 to 30 minutes, until the chocolate has set.

Cut or break the chocolate bark into about 16 pieces. Transfer to a serving dish.

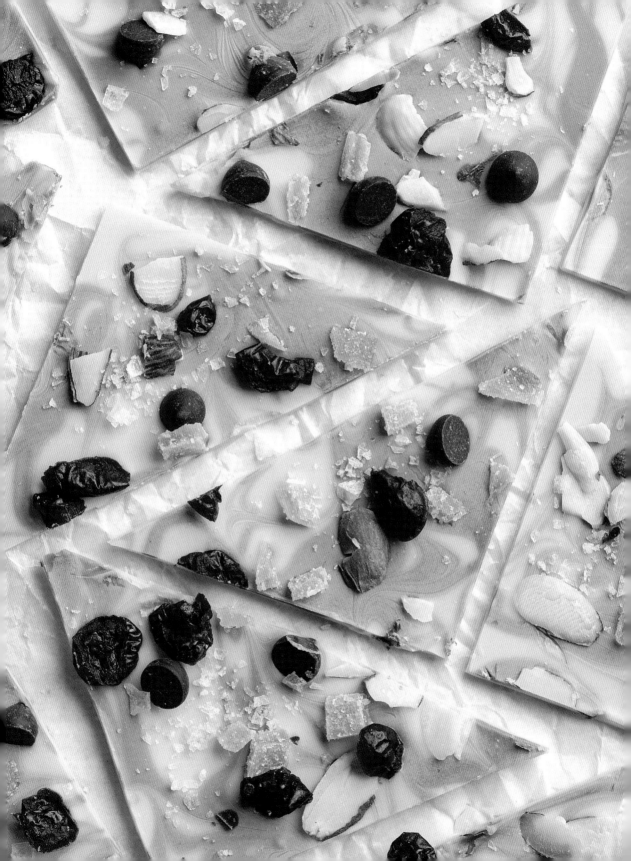

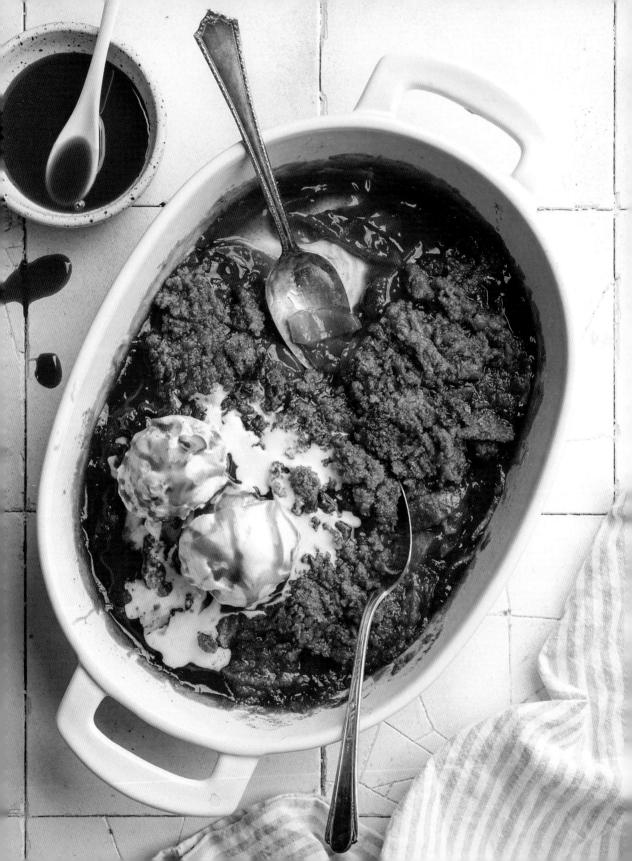

BAKED CARAMEL APPLES

Yield: 7 servings

FILLING

7 apples, Granny Smith or Pink Lady are recommended

1 tbsp (15 ml) lemon juice

1 tsp cinnamon

½ tsp salt

2 tbsp (16 g) whole wheat flour

1 cup (220 g) brown sugar

TOPPING

½ cup (113 g) butter, chopped into small pieces

1 tsp cinnamon

½ cup (100 g) granulated sugar

½ cup (110 g) brown sugar

⅓ cup (40 g) whole wheat flour

Vanilla ice cream (optional)

Apples provide dietary fiber and polyphenol compounds that partner with gut microbes to create an environment that may help to reduce the risk of cancer. Observational population studies link apples with a lower risk of the estrogen receptor negative (ER-) form of breast cancer. Here is another quick and fun way to prepare apples for a more nutritious snack option: Spread apple slices with peanut butter, as this will satisfy hunger longer than other lower-fiber snacks.

Preheat the oven to 350°F (180°C). Core the apples and cut into ¼-inch (6-mm) slices, then cut those slices in half widthwise.

In a large bowl, combine the apples and all the filling ingredients. Stir well and transfer to a 13 x 9–inch (23 x 33–cm) baking dish.

In a separate bowl, combine the topping ingredients, and mash them together with a fork until the mixture forms small- and medium-sized clumps.

Sprinkle the topping evenly over the apples.

Bake for 40 to 45 minutes, or until the liquid has thickened and the apples are tender. Cool for 10 minutes and serve with a scoop of vanilla ice cream, if using.

TROPICAL FRUIT SALAD WITH CITRUS POPPY SEED DRESSING

Yield: 12 servings

DRESSING

1 medium lemon

1 lime

2 mandarin oranges

¼ cup (60 ml) honey

½ tsp ginger paste, or grated fresh ginger

½ tsp poppy seeds

SALAD

10 mandarin oranges, peeled, sectioned

2 cups (332 g) strawberries, sliced

5 kiwis, sliced

1 pineapple, peeled, cored, cut into bite-sized chunks

3 mangoes, peeled, pitted, cut into bite-sized chunks

Fruit salads are a pretty reliable sign of spring and warmer weather around our house. We love fruit! We eat it year-round, but come spring our counters and refrigerator are packed with fresh fruit. I use a few special ingredients that give it a little nuttiness and a touch of zestiness to kick it up a notch. The dressing is truly magical. The combination of citrus juices with honey is phenomenal in the fruit salad dressing. This fresh fruit salad is fabulous with whatever you have on hand. I love carambola (star fruit) and papaya in this salad as well.

To make the dressing: Wash and dry the lemon, lime and mandarin oranges. Zest the washed and dried citrus with a zester or fine grater. Add to either an 8-ounce (240-ml) measuring cup or small bowl. Cut each fruit in half, and squeeze the juice into the measuring cup. (You should get about ½ cup [120 ml] of juice.)

Add the honey, ginger and poppy seeds to the juice mixture, and whisk until combined. Set aside, or cover and refrigerate if serving more than one day later.

For the fruit salad: Place the fruit in a large bowl. Pour the dressing on top and toss to coat. Refrigerate for about 30 minutes before serving.

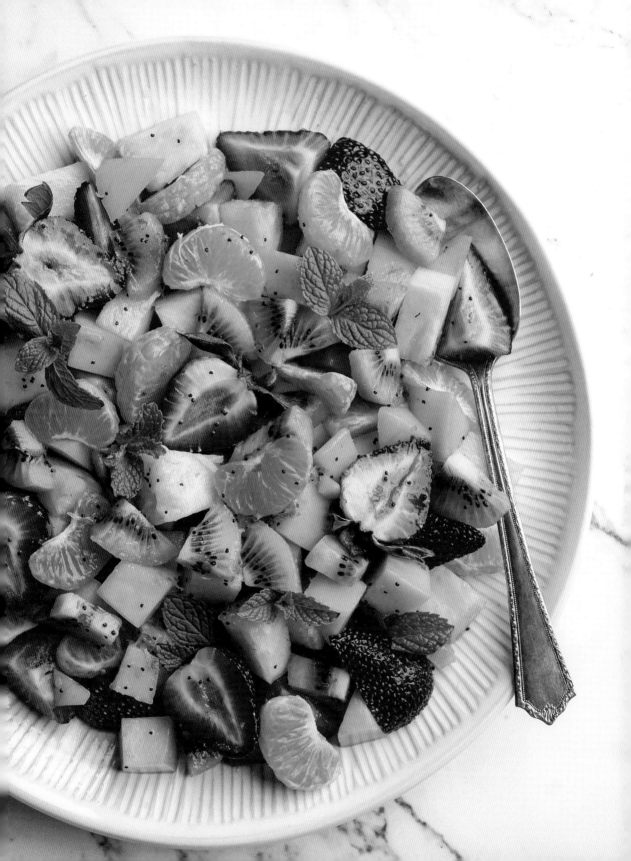

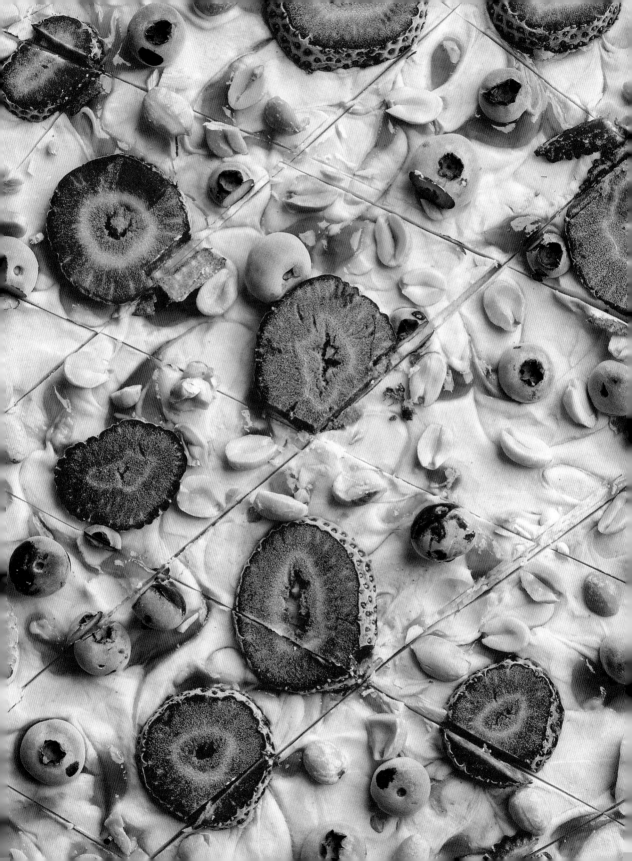

PEANUT BUTTER AND BERRY FROZEN YOGURT BARK

Yield: 8 servings

2–2½ cups (480–600 ml) Greek yogurt, vanilla or plain

2 tbsp (30 ml) honey

½ cup (129 g) peanut butter

3–4 tbsp (60–80 g) strawberry jam

¾ cup (94 g) strawberries, quartered

¼ cup (37 g) blueberries

½ cup (73 g) peanuts, low sodium

You will love how easy to make this Peanut Butter and Berry Frozen Yogurt Bark is. Made with creamy peanut butter and Greek yogurt and topped with fresh fruit and peanuts, this bark makes for a delicious and nutritious snack or dessert! Peanuts don't have just one nutrient that can help in preventing cancer: They have many! Some of these include unsaturated fats and healthy vitamins and minerals, all of which have cancer-preventing qualities. One serving equals approximately ⅓ cup (30 grams) or one handful of nuts. Since all nuts have a similar nutrient content, a wide variety of them can be included as part of a healthy diet to support reducing cancer risk.

Add the yogurt, honey and peanut butter to a large bowl. Mix until it is combined to your liking.

Spread the mixture in an even layer on a lined sheet pan (I use a quarter sheet pan).

Cover the pan with plastic wrap and transfer it to the freezer. Freeze for 4 hours, or until firm.

When ready to eat, break the bark or use a knife to cut the bark into the size of your choice.

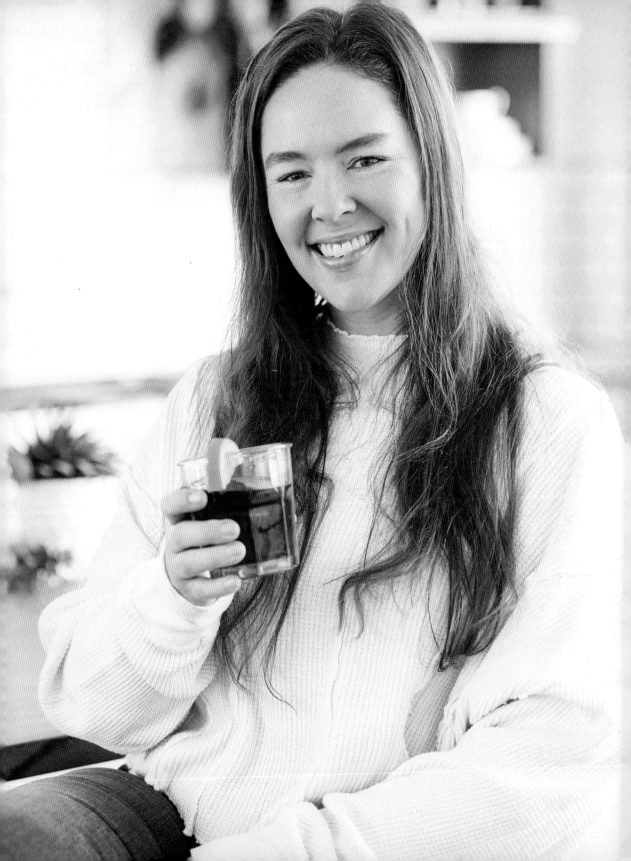

Mocktails
WITHOUT THE RISK

Mocktails mimic alcoholic cocktails, but because they are alcohol-free, you can drink them without any worry of increasing cancer risk! Cheers to that! Non-Alcoholic Sangria (page 146), Ginger and Turmeric Hot Cider (page 141), Watermelon Granita with Minty Basil Syrup Mocktail (page 148)—you name it, they can be made sans booze. Spritzers work especially well as mocktails and can be made with a variety of ingredients, plus fruit and juice. Another great thing about mocktails? They can be made as big batches ahead of time and are ready to serve if you have company coming. Plus mocktails are perfect for kids! Whether you are in the mood for a light cool drink, a warm Matcha Latte (page 142) or a Turmeric Latte (page 139), you will be able to enjoy these drinks and know they are supporting a cancer-prevention lifestyle!

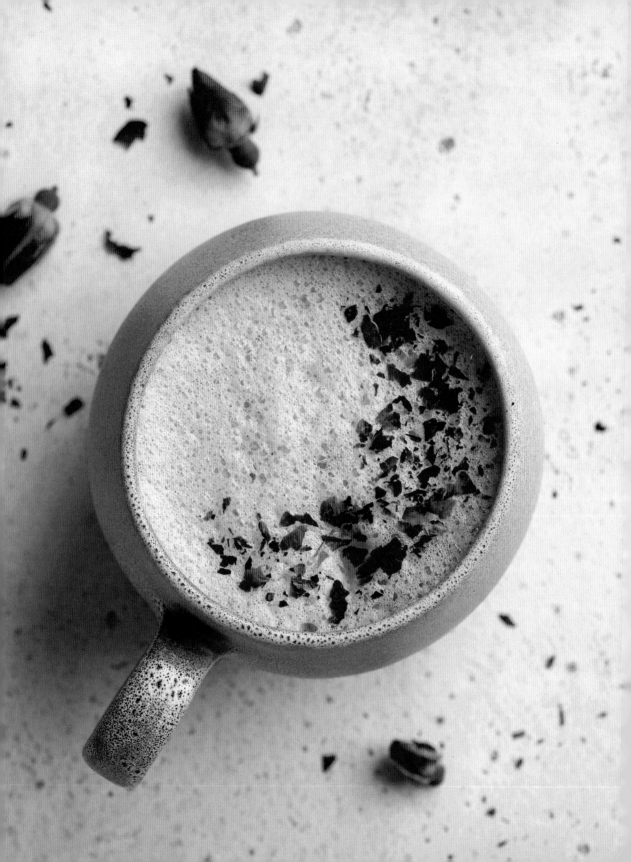

TURMERIC LATTE

Yield : 2 servings

1 ½ cup (360 ml) milk of your choice
¼ tsp turmeric, powder or grated root
¼ tsp ginger
¼ tsp cinnamon, plus more for serving
½ tsp vanilla extract
1 tsp maple syrup
Dash of black pepper

Jazz up breakfast, or any latte break time, with this golden latte. Studies suggest that ginger and the curcumin in turmeric have anti-inflammatory and antioxidant effects. These benefits come from the spices in their root form or dried and ground in spice-jar form—not in pill form. Fresh, unprocessed food sources are different from ginger or turmeric dietary supplements. There is little research to ensure turmeric or curcumin pills or other supplements are safe when used in combination with cancer treatments, including surgery, radiation and chemotherapy. Make sure to enjoy this fun spice in edible form from the grocery store.

Put all the ingredients in a saucepan, and whisk constantly over a gentle heat, ideally with a milk frother if you have one. Once hot, pour into mugs and sprinkle with a little more cinnamon to serve.

GINGER PINK LEMONADE

Yield: 4 servings

2½ cups (600 ml) water

1-inch (2.5-cm) piece of fresh ginger, peeled

2 tbsp (30 ml) agave nectar

¾ cup (125 g) sliced raspberries or strawberries, fresh or frozen

¾ cup (180 ml) freshly squeezed lemon juice (about 6 medium lemons)

Ice cubes

The spicy sweetness of ginger pairs beautifully in a tart lemonade, softened with red berries that lend a pretty pink shade and sweet flavor. With only a touch of agave nectar, the berries offer the bulk of the natural sweetness to complement lemons in this thirst-quenching beverage. It is as beautiful as it is delicious. Serve a single glass over ice, in pitchers at parties, at a picnic on a sunny day or keep it in the fridge for up to 7 days for a healthy hydration option.

Add the water, ginger, agave, berries and freshly squeezed lemon juice to the jar of a large blender. Process for a few seconds, until smooth. Transfer it to a pitcher and store in the refrigerator until serving time. Fill four large glasses with ice, and serve.

GINGER AND TURMERIC HOT CIDER

Yield: 1 serving

1 cup (240 ml) fresh sweet apple cider

1 tsp grated fresh ginger

1 tsp grated fresh turmeric

1 strip (½ x ½ inch [1.3 x 1.3 cm]) lemon peel, white part (albedo) included

Dash of cinnamon (optional)

Warm apple cider is the perfect winter comfort drink. This special version combines two potent spices, ginger and turmeric, for a unique flavor and nutrition profile. Fresh ginger, for example, contains a pungent substance called gingerol, while turmeric gets it characteristic yellow hue from the class of cancer-fighting compounds called curcuminoids. Both are being studied for their anti-inflammatory and antioxidant properties.

In a small saucepan, combine the cider, ginger, turmeric and lemon peel. Over medium-high heat, warm until a ring of bubbles appears around the edge of the pan, about 3 minutes.

Cover the pan and let it steep for 5 minutes.

Pour the cider through a tea strainer into a mug and add a dash of cinnamon, if using. Serve immediately.

MATCHA LATTE

Yield: 1 serving

½–1 tsp matcha powder

¼ cup (60 ml) hot water, plus more as needed

¼ cup (60 ml) warmed coconut milk, or milk of your choice, plus more as needed

Maple syrup, honey, stevia or other sweetener of your choice, to taste (optional)

Matcha powder is made from ground green tea leaves. Unlike when you drink steeped green tea, you consume the entire tea leaf in a matcha latte. Matcha contains the nutrients from the entire tea leaf, which results in a greater amount of caffeine, catechins and antioxidants than typically found in green tea. Matcha is rich in catechins, a class of plant compounds in tea that act as natural antioxidants. Antioxidants help stabilize harmful free radicals, which are compounds that can damage cells and cause chronic disease.

Sift your matcha so it is lump-free. Spoon the matcha into a large mug. Add the hot water and whisk briskly, in an up and down motion, until frothy—about 30 seconds or so. Add the milk and whisk until well combined.

Taste and add additional water, coconut milk and/or sweetener to your liking, if using.

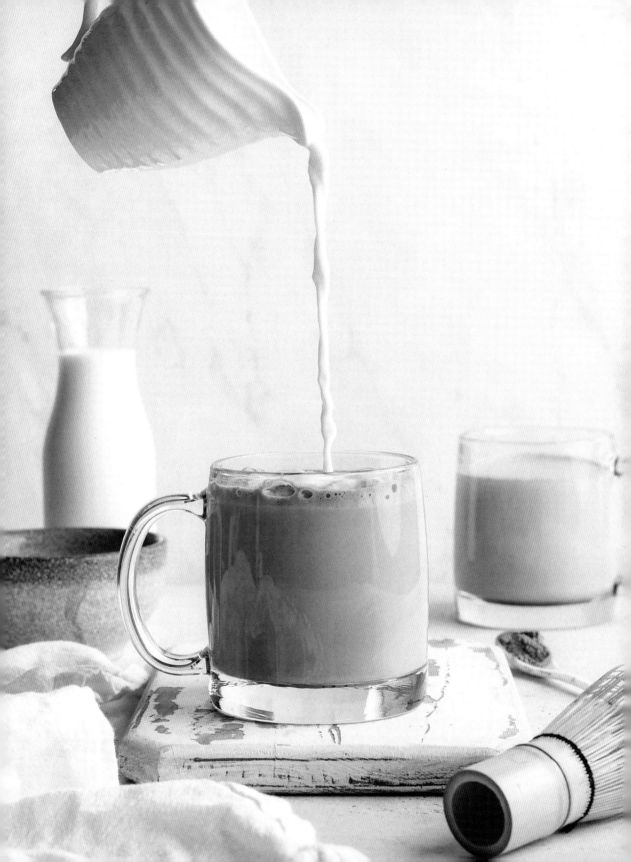

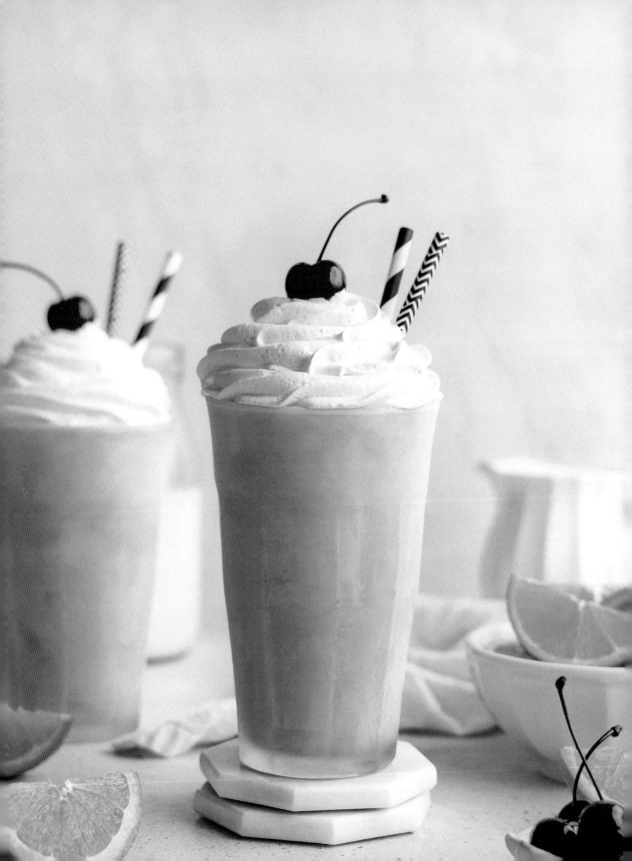

ORANGE CREAMSICLE SHAKE

Yield : 2 servings

¾ cup (180 ml) orange soda

2 scoops of vanilla ice cream

2 scoops of orange sherbet

3 tbsp (6 g) whipped cream, for topping

Orange slice and a Maraschino cherry, for garnish (optional)

An Orange Creamsicle Shake is a yummy mix of creamy vanilla with a punch of orange soda. This milkshake is a classic flavor combo that everyone just adores. Homemade milkshakes are so fun to make, and they cost just a fraction of what they do at a restaurant. Especially in the warmer months of the year, my kids and I like to shop for new ingredients and come up with new milkshake recipes. This orange creamsicle one might just be our favorite!

Add the orange soda, vanilla ice cream and orange sherbet to a blender and blend until frothy. Pour it into two 12-ounce (355-ml) glasses, and top with whipped cream. Garnish with the orange slice and the cherry, if using.

NON-ALCOHOLIC SANGRIA

Yield: 6 servings

1 lemon, sliced

1 lime, sliced

Fresh orange slices

½ cup (50 g) cranberries

2 cups (480 ml) cranberry juice

2 cups (480 ml) grape juice

1 cup (240 ml) orange juice, with pulp

½ cup (120 ml) lemon juice

4 cups (960 ml) sparkling mineral water (or lemon-lime soda)

This Non-alcoholic Sangria is loaded with cancer-prevention power! The cancer-protective potential of cranberries comes primarily from a package of phenolic compounds. Because many of these compounds are complex molecules broken down by gut microbes, there is potential for broad, beneficial effects on the gut microbiota and the reduction of inflammation. Balance the fresh cranberries' tartness by mixing them with other fruits, such as oranges, apples and pears, for a relish or salsa.

In a large pitcher, add the lemon slices, lime slices, orange slices and cranberries. Add the cranberry juice, grape juice, orange juice and lemon juice. Stir well.

Refrigerate until ready to use. Just before serving, add the sparkling mineral water or lemon-lime soda. Mix well.

* See image on page 136.

VIRGIN MARY MOCKTAIL

Yield : 1 serving

3 oz (89 ml) low-sodium tomato juice
1 tbsp (15 ml) lemon juice
Dash of Worcestershire sauce
Freshly ground black pepper, to taste
2 dashes of hot sauce, or to taste
1 celery rib, for garnish (optional)
1 pickle spear, for garnish (optional)
3 green olives, for garnish (optional)

Making a Virgin Mary Mocktail is as easy as removing the vodka from your favorite Bloody Mary recipe and substituting it with this easy, flavorful recipe. Use it as a brunch drink, a mocktail for baby showers or as a cooling non-alcoholic aperitif during hot summer days.

In a cocktail shaker, mix the tomato juice and lemon juice. Pour the mixture into a highball glass filled with ice cubes. Add the Worcestershire sauce, pepper and hot sauce to taste. Garnish with the celery rib, pickle spear and olives, if using.

WATERMELON GRANITA WITH MINTY BASIL SYRUP MOCKTAIL

Yield: 4 servings

GRANITA

4 cups (608 g) cubed watermelon

¼ cup (60 ml) fresh lime juice (2 to 3 limes)

1 cup (240 ml) preferred flavor of soda water, chilled

Mint and basil leaves, for garnishing

SYRUP

½ cup (46 g) mint leaves

½ cup (12 g) basil leaves

1 cup (240 ml) water

½ cup (120 ml) honey

Indulgent without the guilt, this frozen mocktail is a refreshing way to cool off! The granita on its own is a bit tart, so make sure to add the minty basil syrup! Dietary antioxidants in watermelon, such as vitamin C, may help prevent cancer by combatting free radicals. Some studies have also linked lycopene intake with a lower risk of prostate cancer.

Place the watermelon in a food processor, and add the lime juice. Pulse until just combined. Pour the mixture through a strainer over a 9 x 13–inch (23 x 33–cm) freezer-safe baking dish.

Transfer the dish to the freezer, and let the mixture chill for about 30 minutes.

Scrape the watermelon into smaller bits using one or two forks, and then return the dish to the freezer for another half hour. Repeat the process three to four more times, or until the granita is completely frozen.

Meanwhile, make the syrup by combining the mint, basil, water and honey in a small saucepan. Bring it to a low simmer, and cook for about 10 minutes, stirring until the honey has dissolved. Remove it from the heat and let it cool completely. Strain it into a glass jar. To assemble the mocktail, scoop the granita into four 12-ounce (355-ml) glasses. Drizzle with 2 or 3 tablespoons (30 to 45 ml) of the syrup, then top with the chilled soda water.

Garnish with additional basil and mint leaves. Serve with a small spoon or straw.

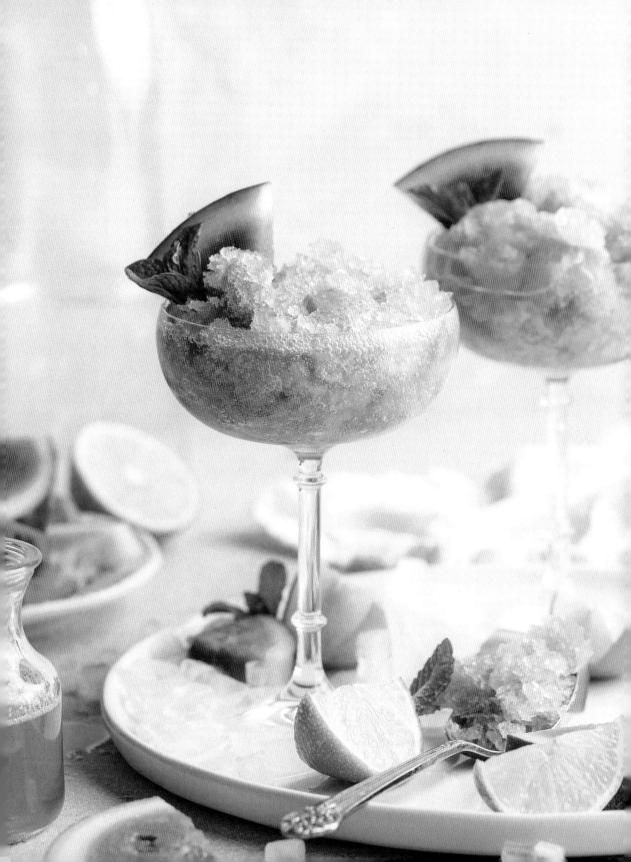

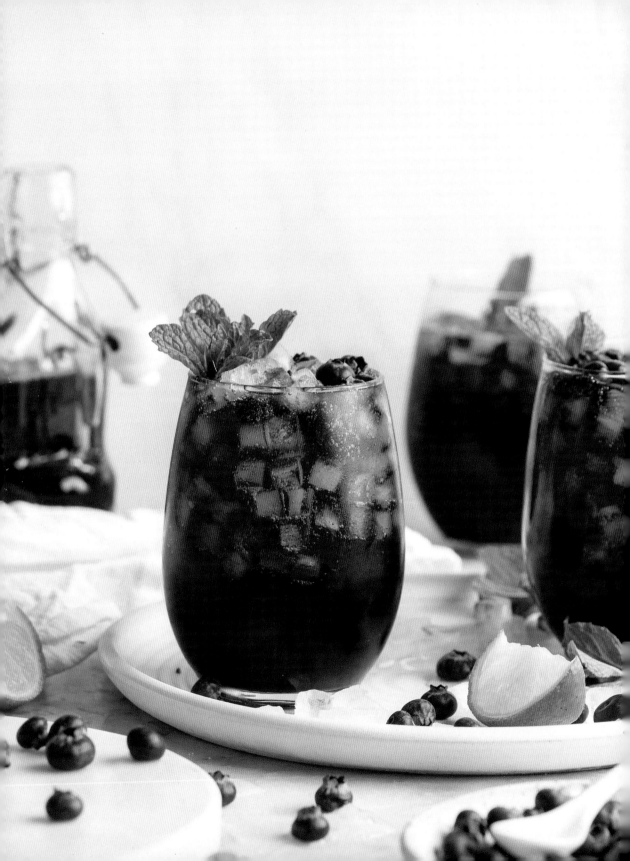

BLUEBERRY-GINGER COOLER

Yield : 8 servings

34 oz (1 L) water

1¼ cups (185 g) fresh blueberries, plus more for garnishing

1 heaping tbsp (6 g) grated ginger

4–5 tbsp (60–75 g) granulated sugar, adjust amount to taste

Ice cubes

3 (12-oz [355-ml]) cans of lemon-lime sparkling water, unsweetened

Mint leaves, for garnish

Blueberries, rich in protective plant compounds, may improve brain, eye and heart health along with reducing cancer risk. And ginger has anti-inflammatory properties that relieve swelling. The serving size of blueberries is about ½ cup (74 g).

To a pan on medium-high heat, add the water, blueberries and grated ginger. Let it all come to a boil. Once the mixture starts boiling, add the sugar and mix until it dissolves.

Now lower the heat and, using the back of your spatula, mash the blueberries. Mash all of them and let the mixture simmer for another 10 to 15 minutes. Remove it from the heat, and once the syrup has cooled down, cover it with cling wrap, and let it sit at room temperature for 2 to 3 hours. This is important so that the flavors mix in well.

After 2 to 3 hours have elapsed, strain the syrup into a clear bowl. At this point you can cover it and keep it refrigerated until ready to use. To serve the blueberry-ginger cooler, fill two-thirds of a 12-ounce (355-ml) glass with the syrup, and add ice cubes. Then add lemon-lime sparkling water, and stir so that the soda and syrup combine well. Garnish with mint leaves and fresh blueberries.

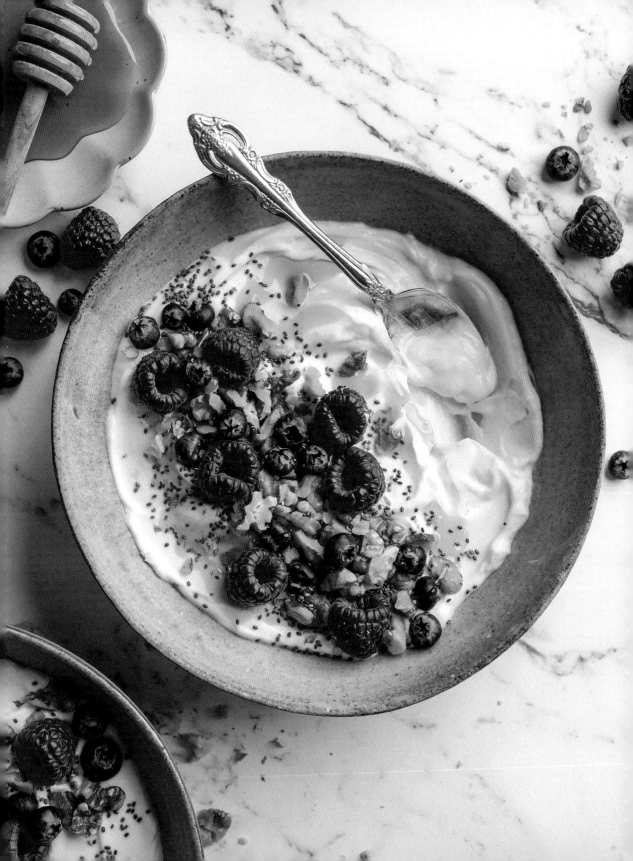

ACKNOWLEDGMENTS

Thanks to everyone on the Page Street Publishing team who helped me so much. Special thanks to Marissa Giambelluca, the ever-awesome editorial director, and Meg Baskis, the amazing creative director and the greatest cover designer I could ever imagine!

Huge shout-out to the incredible photographers Mark Cornellison and Amie MacGregor, who did their magic to bring this book to even more life with photography!

I am so grateful to the amazing communities of eager and motivated cancer survivors across my social media pages: Thank you for sharing your goals, stories, hardships and joys with me. It means the world to be here to support you and be supported back!

And of course, lots of love to my three amazing children, who cheered me on each step of the way while I wrote this fun and supportive book for so many cancer survivors to use and enjoy.

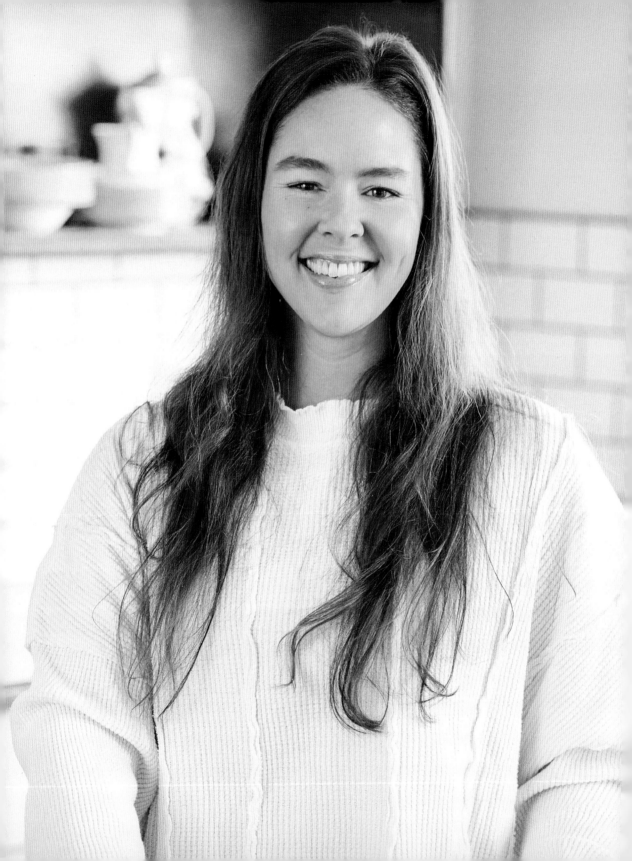

ABOUT THE AUTHOR

Nichole Andrews, "the Oncology Dietitian," has worked with adult and pediatric cancer survivors of all stages for over ten years. As a private practicing oncology dietitian, she has served thousands of cancer survivors in one-of-a-kind, empowering, simplified cancer nutrition and lifestyle programs. She is also the creator of acclaimed cancer nutrition and private lifestyle coaching, group coaching programs, menus, supportive courses, customized exercise programs and more. These initiatives have helped cancer survivors go from being unsure about nutrition to being confident with food and energized to live a life they are excited about.

After Nichole had worked in different areas of the clinical setting to support survivors, she quickly realized that the misinforming cancer nutrition advice was not slowing down, and new cancer survivors kept falling victim to these outlandish and dangerous diet trends, supplements and claims regarding cancer nutrition. Understandably, cancer survivors were just trying to do their best and beat cancer. Nichole decided to take significant action to stop the fearmongering and confusion. She took to social media, where she has continued to provide credible information and science-backed advice, building an active and supportive community of tens of thousands of people.

CONNECT WITH NICHOLE:

Website: theoncologydietitian.com

Instagram: @oncology.nutrition.rd

TikTok: @oncology.nutrition.rd

Facebook: Nichole Andrews, RDN

INDEX